Praise fc
Psych

MW01504099

"Bravo! I love the question-and-answer format because it sounds like a conversation in my office. As a parent and a child and adolescent psychiatrist, I have tried to navigate the careful terrain of supporting parents and children in decisions about whether to treat psychiatric conditions with medication— Drs. Kolevzon, Jaffe, and Trelles have done a marvelous job in achieving this goal. *A Parent's Guide to Starting Psychiatric Medications for Kids* will be an important resource."

—Victor Fornari, MD
Vice Chair for Child and Adolescent Psychiatry
Zucker School of Medicine at Hofstra/Northwell

"Parents, adolescents, curious children, pediatricians, child and adolescent psychiatrists, and trainees from many medical disciplines: when you open *A Parent's Guide to Starting Psychiatric Medications for Kids*, you will probably feel relief and excitement that this book exists. You will also realize how essential it is to be a highly informed parent or an ideal prescriber. This guide is an engaging resource filled with clear answers to questions that parents often wish their providers addressed systematically, even when time is limited. It also specifically addresses medication, which is a crucial aspect of child and adolescent psychiatry treatment that is often the most distressing and the least understood by families. It is a beautifully practical approach to the very real possibility of fear and stigma overshadowing reality when it comes to this topic. This accomplishment is particularly significant given the urgent need for solutions to common challenges in delivering care as we navigate the current epidemic of child mental health needs."

—Anne L. Glowinski, MD, MPE
Robert Porter Distinguished Professor in Child and Adolescent
Psychiatry and Behavioral Sciences, University of California San Francisco

"When looking for trustworthy information on psychiatric medications for their children, parents often have to wade through stigmatized views, advice from well-wishers, and direct-to-consumer advertising. Bucking this trend, *A Parent's Guide to Starting Psychiatric Medications for Kids* provides a new resource that is as approachable as it is comprehensive, as compassionate as it is evidence-based—in short, a book full of light, in a space so often consumed by heat."

—Andrés Martin, MD, PhD
Riva Ariella Ritvo Professor, Child Study Center, Yale School of Medicine

"Taking a no-nonsense approach, *A Parent's Guide to Starting Psychiatric Medications for Kids* answers parents' most common and anxiety-provoking questions about treating their children with psychiatric medications in an evidence-based, gentle, and often humorous manner. Reading this book feels a lot like sitting around the dinner table with these kindhearted and compassionate authors, whose fine book I will certainly recommend to families."

—Jess P. Shatkin, MD, MPH
Vice Chair for Education & Professor, Department of Child & Adolescent Psychiatry, NYU Grossman School of Medicine

"As the parent of a profoundly autistic son with a history of very aggressive and self-injurious behavior, I know firsthand the challenges of finding the right psychiatric care. *A Parent's Guide to Starting Psychiatric Medications for Kids* is the guide I wish I had—offering practical, compassionate, and evidence-based advice to help families navigate tough decisions with confidence and hope."

—Amy S. F. Lutz, PhD
Vice President, National Council on Severe Autism

"Finally!! This is the book I wish I had when we first considered medication for my daughter with autism. Parents shouldn't need a medical degree to understand their child's medical options. And now they don't!"

"Have you ever wished that you could have all the time you need with your provider to ask every question you might have about psychiatric medication for your child? And wouldn't it be wonderful if the provider answered knowledgeably with clear, honest explanations, in a comfortable conversational tone, with humanity and kindness? This is your book! The authors are friendly expert guides who know the territory and are down-to-earth communicators."

FAMILIUS

Published by Familius LLC, www.familius.com
PO Box 1130, Sanger, CA 93657

Familius books are available at special discounts for bulk purchases, whether for
sales promotions or for family or corporate use. For more information, contact
Familius Sales at orders@familius.com.

Library of Congress Control Number: 2024946874

Print ISBN 9798893960457
Ebook ISBN 9798893965124

Printed in China

Edited by Peg Sandkam and Mikaela Sircable
Cover and book design by Brooke Jorden

10 9 8 7 6 5 4 3 2 1

First Edition

A Parent's Guide to Starting

Psychiatric Medications for Kids

Start Low and Go Slow
When Medicating Children

ALEXANDER KOLEVZON, MD   ROBERT JAFFE, MD   PILAR TRELLES, MD

Brief Biographies

Who Are We?

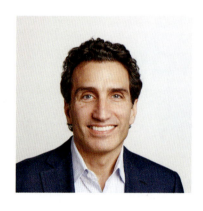

Alex Kolevzon, MD, is a child and adolescent psychiatrist with more than twenty years of clinical and research experience. He is a Professor of Psychiatry and Pediatrics at the Icahn School of Medicine at Mount Sinai in New York, where he serves as the Clinical Director of the Seaver Autism Center for Research and Treatment. His research is focused on developing new treatments for people with neurodevelopmental disorders, which include behavioral interventions, medications, and gene therapy. He is also the Director of Child and Adolescent Psychiatry for the Mount Sinai Health System. In this role, Alex is dedicated to ensuring children, adolescents, and families across New York City receive the best possible care from experts at Mount Sinai, advancing science across childhood psychiatric disorders, and training the next generation of clinicians specializing in children's mental health. Alex is also passionate about education; he is a frequently invited speaker nationally and internationally and has won numerous awards as an active teacher, mentor, and clinical supervisor. Alex has also written three books for medical students and residents in general psychiatry and is a coauthor of the *Textbook of Autism Spectrum Disorders*. This is Alex's first book for families and the compilation of discussions with thousands of caregivers struggling with the decision of whether or not to use psychiatric medication for their children.

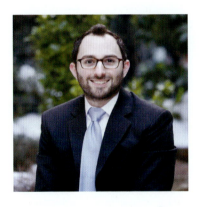

Robbie Jaffe, MD, is an Associate Professor of Psychiatry and Pediatrics at the Icahn School of Medicine at Mount Sinai, where he is the Training Director for Child and Adolescent Psychiatry. Robbie teaches the psychiatrists of tomorrow as the Program Director for Mount Sinai's Child and Adolescent Psychiatry Fellowship. Robbie runs a teaching clinic working with a team of fellows, psychologists, and social workers to help kids and teens with anxiety, obsessive-compulsive disorder (OCD), and tics and Tourette's disorder. He is also the Director of the Tourette Association of America's Center of Excellence at Mount Sinai, where he researches novel treatments for Tourette's disorder and attention-deficit/hyperactivity disorder (ADHD). He has written chapters and given invited lectures on tic disorders and how they interact with anxiety, OCD, and ADHD. Most of all, Robbie loves to both teach and help patients and their loved ones and is humbled to provide families with this resource.

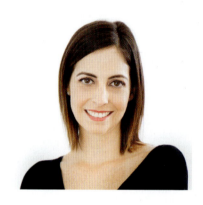

Pilar Trelles, MD, is a native Peruvian but spent twenty years in the New York City area, where she completed her postgraduate training in general psychiatry at Rutgers New Jersey Medical School and child and adolescent psychiatry at the Icahn School of Medicine at Mount Sinai. After child psychiatry training, she pursued an additional specialized fellowship in neurodevelopmental disorders, also at Mount Sinai, where she focused on using genetics to advance therapeutics in the field. She is currently faculty at Harvard Medical School and works at Boston Children's Hospital, where she leads psychiatric care for children with autism spectrum disorder and efforts to increase diversity and inclusion in psychiatric clinical trials more broadly. Pilar is passionate about working with caregivers and other stakeholders to bridge advances in the field of child psychiatry to community care, and she has participated in multiple research projects and educational initiatives with this goal in mind. Pilar is also invested in medical education and is a frequently invited speaker in national and international meetings.

Contents

Preface

Why Are We Writing This Guide?

A Parent's Guide to Starting Psychiatric Medications for Kids was inspired by discussions we have had with thousands of parents about whether or not to use medication to help their children and teens struggling with mental health. All three of us are deeply committed to training and education, and over many years of teaching and collaborating together, it became obvious that caregivers tend to ask many of the same questions and that we all have different, but similar, ways of answering them. The goal of this book is to share our collective knowledge and perspectives on using psychiatric medications in children and adolescents. We review the process of evaluating children and coming to the decision of using psychiatric medications and then discuss different classes of medications in detail. The book is organized in question-and-answer format because this most closely aligns with the decision-making process for caregivers in our experience. The index provides an alphabetical list of all the major topics for ease of use.

We organize medications into broader categories (e.g., antidepressants) and then review different types of medications within those categories (e.g., selective serotonin reuptake inhibitors, or SSRIs) and their uses. We refer to many different medications throughout *A Parent's Guide to Starting Psychiatric Medications for Kids* and discuss those that have specific approval from the United States Food and Drug Administration (FDA) for various childhood psychiatric disorders. We review the differences between "FDA-approved" and "off-label" medications, and each relevant section has tables, which list all the psychiatric medicines that are FDA-approved for children. By convention, we use brand names of medicines because they are more likely to be familiar to caregivers, but the tables list commonly used medications with both the brand and generic names.

For the neuroscientists or pharmacologists among our readers, please understand that we have purposefully (over) simplified what is known about the neurobiology of mental illness and the mechanisms of action of the medicines in order to make the material more accessible to a broad audience.

As academic child psychiatrists, we are all involved in studying new treatments for childhood psychiatric disorders and receive funding from various sources, including the National Institute of Health (NIH), foundations, and, yes, pharmaceutical companies. Alex also consults with various companies that are developing new treatments in neurodevelopmental disorders. While none of us have *actual* conflicts of interest related to this guide, all our sources of funding, consulting activities, and *potential* conflicts of interest are listed in the appendix.

We know that for caregivers, the process of considering psychiatric medications for your child can be a scary one and a path filled with concern and uncertainty. Some caregivers even compare the experience to a battle—a battle of conscience, of judgment, of risks and benefits. It reminds us of a joke where the worried parent is asked if they have any words of wisdom for their child who just enlisted in the Air Force and is about to go to battle. The answer: "Fly low and go slow!"

We hope this guide empowers you to ask your provider all the tough questions to ensure you feel comfortable and confident in your journey of exploring psychiatric medications for your child.

A Historical Perspective

The year is 1820. Joe American, basking in the victory from the War of 1812, comes down with a nasty cough. *Nothing to worry about*, Joe thinks. And why should he? The Industrial Revolution is humming, daylight saving time isn't ruining two weeks each year, and California's rivers are teeming with enough gold that you might even be able to afford housing there. Yes, other than over half the population not being allowed to vote and the lack of Cyber Monday deals, things are good. Real good. Except for ole Joe's cough, which did sometimes bring up some phlegm. And blood. But that's it! Out of an abundance of caution, Joe sees his doctor. Joe's doctor, also named Joe, is a beloved community figure who performs house calls and delivers babies. Dr. Joe pays a visit to Joe and sees that Joe is in markedly more pain than he let on. Dr. Joe isn't burdened with having to choose the right antibiotic—penicillin won't be invented until 1928. Dr. Joe isn't even worried about which likely virus is causing Joe's cough—the germ theory of disease won't gain acceptance until the end of the century. And no, Dr. Joe is not contemplating whether Joe's cough is from tuberculosis, whooping cough, or smoking too many Joe Camels. Dr. Joe only cares that Joe's symptoms are bothering Joe, and he wants to help. Dr. Joe gives Joe an opium tincture. Joe feels a world of relief and is able to get back to his family and live a productive and happy life. Until he dies at thirty-five.

Fortunately, medicine has made many advances since Joe's time. We now know more about the human brain than we ever have in history, which is to say we still know very little about how the brain works. The summation of all of humankind's contributions to studying our minds has resulted in understanding the cause of exactly zero psychiatric conditions. Part of this is tautological, because once a cause is determined, it ceases to be classified as psychiatric. Rett syndrome, for example, was historically a diagnosis in the Diagnostic and Statistical Manual for Mental Disorders (DSM), but it is no longer considered a psychiatric illness now that its genetic cause has been determined (mutations in the *MECP2* gene on the X chromosome). However, common disorders such as depression and anxiety remain a medical mystery. It should be noted that such uncertainty is not without company, even in modern medicine. The cause of high blood pressure (hypertension) is unknown in the overwhelming majority of cases, yet treatments abound to decrease blood pressure and improve health outcomes. To be clear, there have been numerous advances in psychiatry—imaging studies tell us what regions of the brain are implicated, genetic studies have identified hundreds of contributing genes, and we know how alterations in certain chemicals (neurotransmitters) such as serotonin can affect symptoms and their treatment.

The field of child and adolescent psychiatry in particular did not embrace the notion of a biological basis for mental illness until the late 1930s. At that time, the psychiatrist Charles Bradley, quite by accident, discovered that amphetamine (Benzedrine) improved social, academic, and emotional functioning in children with severe behavioral disturbances. His observations are the first evidence of the benefit of using a stimulant medication to treat what we now call attention-deficit/hyperactivity disorder (ADHD). Since then, the field has advanced significantly, and the relative safety and benefits of many different medications have been established through rigorous research studies. Today, clinicians now have a robust evidence base to rely on in determining treatment options for children with psychiatric disorders, as well as established treatment guidelines from professional organizations, such as the American Academy of Child and Adolescent Psychiatry.

We're not always in favor of medication. Really. In fact, it is only in the past half-century that medications allowed psychiatrists to move away from psychotherapy in the first place. So why do we prescribe them? Simply put, because they can be undeniably helpful. We know much more about human physiology today than Dr. Joe did. But like Dr. Joe, the current practice of psychiatry remains focused on reducing symptoms. While not curative, psychiatric medications can be highly effective and enable people to dramatically improve their quality of life.

We wrote this book because after years of prescribing to thousands of patients, certain questions come up time and again. Families want to learn about medications. Also, it turns out that not everything on the internet is true. Our aim is one resource (which our lawyers have reiterated is not a substitute for medical advice) where families can turn for good (but not legally binding) information on common psychiatric medications they or their loved ones might be prescribed (by their legally responsible physician).

Understanding medications, how they are organized into various categories (or "classes"), and their role in addressing symptoms is complicated and convoluted. Medications generally help with specific symptoms (like excessive worrying), yet get approval by the Food and Drug Administration (FDA) for specific disorders (like generalized anxiety disorder). Ritalin is approved for use in ADHD but improves focus. Medications also all belong to a class, mainly determined by what it was initially used to treat. For example, Prozac is in the antidepressant class because it was first used in depression. But Prozac also helps with anxiety and obsessive-compulsive disorder (OCD). Abilify is an antipsychotic because it helps with hallucinations. Abilify also helps with irritability associated with autism spectrum disorder. And depression. And bipolar disorder. And Tourette's disorder. Yet Abilify is classified as an antipsychotic. Confused? Hopefully this will all become clear, or at least a little bit clearer, as you read on.

With this context in mind, *A Parent's Guide to Starting Psychiatric Medications for Kids* is organized by medication class rather than diagnosis because the same medication may be used across many diagnoses. This organization is designed to make it easier to search for specific medications (see the tables and index). For each medication, we will also note which disorders it is commonly prescribed for so you know the medication options for a given diagnosis.

Chapter 1

Approach to Treatment

Deciding whether to start your child on a medication can be a difficult decision. For some issues, like a urinary tract infection, the decision to medicate might take only a second. You have objective symptoms even Dr. Joe can detect and today are supported by a laboratory test that can confirm the diagnosis and even determine the best antibiotic for treatment. In other instances, however, the decision can be much more complicated. With mental health, symptoms can be more subjective and difficult to detect and understand. Often stigma leads to reluctance to fully reveal symptoms or seek care altogether. Mental health problems during childhood and adolescence are especially challenging to diagnose and treat; kids are in the throes of rapid developmental changes and societal expectations are shifting dramatically under their growing bodies.

We imagine that if you are reading this book, this is something you are exploring or a road that you already started traveling. You may also be observing changes in the behavior of your child, including emotional distress, social problems, or academic challenges. They may be having difficulties in their daily functioning, in making friends or learning, or even just in getting a good night's sleep. There are many potential "first signs" warning of mental health problems for families. And maybe there have only been small concerns over the years that have amassed to the point where now you feel a crisis is looming. For many families, it's a crisis that forces them to consider medicine.

As you venture down this road, the most important thing is to have a thorough assessment and clearly identify the symptoms you want to treat. We say "symptoms" purposefully because despite all the studies, fancy names of disorders in the DSM, and advances in understanding biology, psychiatry today continues to treat symptoms and not diagnostic labels. While it is very appealing to seek out or receive a specific "diagnosis," often kids did not read the diagnostic manual and present with a broad constellation of symptoms that do not fit neatly into one category. Once symptoms are distressing and disruptive, it may be time to consider medicine. The decision should be collaborative, ideally between you as the caregiver/s, the child, and the provider. Children may be at various stages of readiness to participate in this conversation, but your doctor should seem well-informed, be thoughtful, and be able to communicate their thinking clearly to help you make the most informed decision.

Sticking to the basics of a thorough evaluation and listening very carefully, like Dr. Joe, is expected and the best path forward in determining appropriate treatment. Once that assessment is made and symptoms are prioritized, be sure to ask lots of questions if medication is being recommended. In this guidebook, we answer all the questions most commonly asked by parents and caregivers over our collective experience. *A Parent's Guide to Starting Psychiatric Medications for Kids* is intended as a general guide to assist you in taking this important step of using psychiatric medication to help your child.

Medication Development Process

Figure 1

Pre-Clinical

Testing on animals for toxicity.

INVESTIGATIONAL NEW DRUG (IND) APPLICATION.

Describes the manufacturer's plans for testing the drug in clinical trials. If approved by the FDA, the manufacturer becomes the sponsor of an IND.

Clinical Trials

PHASE I

Clinical trials test for safety and dosing ranges.

20–80 patients; approximately 60% move to Phase II.

PHASE II

Clinical trials test for efficacy in the patients that the drug is intended to treat.

From a few dozen to hundreds of patients; approximately 30% move to Phase III.

PHASE III

Clinical trials test for efficacy in the patients that the drug is intended to treat.

100s–1000s of patients; approximately 60% move to the new drug application process.

Review & Approval Process

NEW DRUG APPLICATION REVIEW

Once the drug has successfully completed the Phase III trials, the manufacturer generally submits a new drug application to the FDA. Approximately 85% are approved.

FDA APPROVAL RESULTS

FDA either approves or denies approval for the drug for marketing and sales in the U.S.

Chapter 2

General Questions

What does the process of getting medicines approved for children look like?

This is such a critical question and the basis for everything else we will review in this book. For medications to be commercially available and dispensed by a pharmacy, they need to undergo extensive testing and ongoing monitoring for safety by the FDA (figure 1). There are many stages for medications to get approval by the FDA; testing usually begins in animals (preclinical) before healthy humans (Phase I) to assess safety. Next are Phase II trials, which are small studies in humans who have the condition the medication is supposed to help (e.g., depression). If the medication is safe and effective in Phase II studies, testing moves on to Phase III, which involves a larger number of participants with the condition, rigorous methods (e.g., placebo control group), and testing across multiple sites. In general, two Phase III studies (known as registration trials) are needed to demonstrate safety and efficacy for the FDA to grant approval. Finally, Phase IV studies continue to evaluate the long-term risks and benefits of a medication after it is already on the market.

What about unknown risks or problems that are only obvious after many years?

The long-term benefits of successfully treating emotional and behavioral health disorders profoundly outweigh the risks of not treating, which could include low self-esteem, school failure, substance use, relationship problems, and even suicide. The risk profile of the medications we use is well-established, including in the long term, because most have been approved for at least a decade and used in millions of children to date. Many people are aware of concerning stories about the FDA-approved medications that are only later discovered to have significant previously unknown risks after being available for many years. The risks in the vast majority of these cases became known and led to withdrawal from the market in five years or less. We are aware of only one example of these withdrawn medicines given to children for behavioral reasons—Cylert—for ADHD. Cylert was first available in 1975 but risks of liver toxicity became known after about thirty years and the medication was withdrawn from the market in 2005. Provided a medication has undergone post-marketing surveillance (Phase IV) for a number of years, you should feel confident that the risks are well-known. Simply put, if a medication is on the market for any indication, it has extensive research supporting its safety. Furthermore, the longer it has been out, the better we understand its potential side effects.

Great, so I assume everything that you prescribe has an FDA indication?

Well, sort of. Everything we prescribe has an FDA indication, but not necessarily for the reason it's being prescribed in your child. Every medication has an FDA indication for a very specific group, such as people over eighteen years old with generalized anxiety disorder or children over six years old who have ADHD. Among the challenges we face, relatively few medications are specifically studied in children and adolescents. So while Prozac is FDA-approved to treat OCD in children, among other indications, we also use it to treat other anxiety disorders, like generalized anxiety disorder, where we don't have a specific indication. This is what is known as "off-label" use. Lexapro, on the other hand, received FDA approval in May 2023 to treat generalized anxiety disorder in children and adolescents. While it is tempting to surmise that Lexapro is therefore more effective than Prozac for treating anxiety, this is not necessarily the case. In fact, Prozac and Lexapro basically work the same (selective serotonin reuptake inhibitors) and, while some differences exist, these are unlikely to have a major impact on effectiveness. Instead, the manufacturer of Lexapro (AbbVie) elected to do additional studies in kids to gain the FDA approval, extend their patent, and allow them to market the brand medication. The manufacturer of Prozac (Eli Lilly and Company) did not, but that does not necessarily mean it's less effective. Drug manufacturers are only allowed to market medications for approved uses, so there is a financial incentive to get specific approvals. At the same time, FDA registration trials that qualify for approval (if successful) cost tens of millions of dollars, so these are costly endeavors. And if you've ever experienced insurance denials and seen the out-of-pocket costs for medications, now you have some understanding of why drug companies charge such high prices and why insurance companies do all they can do to avoid paying them.

Why are the FDA approvals so specific?

Let's back up to those Phase III trials. These studies test a specific medication for a particular condition (and often a specific symptom within that condition—like for "irritability associated with autism spectrum disorder") in a specific group of patients. Characteristics for approval go beyond the diagnosis and can include age or sex. Once a medication has two positive large placebo-controlled studies across multiple sites (i.e., Phase III trials), the FDA can grant approval, but only for the particular indication and demographics that were researched in the actual study. If the youngest person in the study was eighteen years old, it won't be approved for kids.

Why don't they just include more kids in the studies?

Mostly because clinical trials are costly in general and more prone to failure in kids for a number of reasons, including the fact that studies in kids are very vulnerable to a high placebo response. High placebo response rates mean that the effect of the medicine has to be very large in order to be significantly different, in statistical terms, from the effect of placebo.

So can you prescribe to a ten-year-old a medication that was approved for ages twelve and up?

Yes, this gets back to the idea of "off-label" use of medication, which is a practice that is common in medicine in general and especially in child psychiatry. From a clinical practice perspective, FDA approval is important, but we have little reason to think that most medicines we prescribe that are safe and effective in twelve-year-olds would not be equally safe and effective in ten-year-olds.

FDA approvals are just one factor in considering which medicine to prescribe. There are many, many studies demonstrating the benefit of medicines we use that don't lead to FDA approvals. Most of the medications we prescribe off-label have been studied and shown to be both safe and effective. It is just that the drug companies did not run them (many of our field's landmark studies were funded by the NIH, so did not submit to the FDA for an approval. As a general rule, we encourage you to discuss all of these considerations with your provider to better understand why they recommend a particular medication and what the alternatives are. This should be part of the same conversations that outline the risks and benefits so you have a full understanding of the options. Throughout this book, we will present information on specific medication classes, along with existing evidence to help you ask the right questions.

Here are a few important concepts and a glossary of terms that will be coming up in the next few chapters.

TABLE 1. GLOSSARY OF TERMS

TERM	DEFINITION
Efficacy	**How well a medication works under the controlled conditions of a clinical trial with respect to specific outcomes.**
Effectiveness	**How well a medication works in "real-world" conditions.**

TERM	DEFINITION
Half-life	The time it takes for the body to eliminate half the concentration of a medication, which typically varies from hours to days, depending on the medicine.
Steady-state	Occurs when the rate of input of a particular medication equals the rate of elimination; typically, steady-state is achieved after four or five half-lives.
Dose	The amount of medication taken at a given time.
Dosage	The frequency of medication administration, which is dependent on the half-life; medication should be administered enough times over the course of the day to allow its concentration to reach a steady state.
Potency	The amount of a medication that allows it to achieve its effect. For example, lower doses of high potency medications are typically needed.
Titration	Slowly increasing medicine over days to months to find the effective dose and dosage.

TERM	DEFINITION
Taper	Gradually reducing medicine to minimize side effects or to discontinue.
Pharmacokinetics	How the body acts on the medication, like rate of absorption and elimination.
Pharmacodynamics	How the medication acts on the body, like blocking serotonin receptors.
Pharmacogenetics	How genes affect the way the body responds to medications.

Chapter 3

Getting to Specifics

Let's say I want to consider medication; what's the process?

Your child would need to have a comprehensive evaluation to establish a diagnosis (or multiple diagnoses) and to identify target symptoms that medicine could potentially address. Evaluations typically consist of time spent with caregivers (depending on the age and developmental level of the child) to discuss the developmental history and present concerns. This is usually followed by meeting your child individually and using a combination of talking, playing, observation, and possibly a physical examination to gather information. Then, the next step is to meet again with you (and your child, depending on their age and developmental level) to discuss impressions and make a plan. Assuming this plan includes medications, this is where your provider would discuss risks, benefits, and alternatives, if any.

Do you ever evaluate a child and not recommend medication?

Great question and the answer has to be considered in the context of the fact that as medication prescribers, most people come to see us to explore medication options, among other goals. Some have waited a long time, perhaps even too long, and are fully ready to start medicine by the time they make the appointment with us. That said, there are cases where we say that medicine probably won't help the symptoms of concern and other cases where we say medicine is absolutely necessary. In many cases, however, medicine will likely help but there may be alternatives and its use can be delayed or potentially avoided. In these cases, it is critical to be able to have a nuanced conversation about risks and benefits with your provider. People bring different biases to using conventional medicine in general. Some want to avoid it at all costs and others are eager to do anything that is safe and effective. We do try and caution caregivers not to let their personal biases affect the well-being of their child given the vast benefits medicine can sometimes provide. What's right for adults to do for themselves may not be the best choice for their child and this is why developing a relationship with a knowledgeable provider whom you trust is so important.

If it was your child, would you medicate them?

If we recommend medicine for your child, we would also give it to ours. And yes, we all have children and have survived, or are actively surviving, their childhood and adolescence.

Won't medications just mask the underlying problem?

While it is true that medications treat symptoms and not diagnostic labels, the symptoms are thought to arise from an underlying disorder and are effectively treated with the medicine. We don't see this as masking an underlying problem or simply applying a band-aid, but instead an effective tool among many that, when applied carefully, can be a critical part of a therapeutic program, including psychotherapy. Psychiatry, like many fields of medicine, has not yet advanced to the development of curative treatments. However, our goal is symptom remission—or at least significant symptomatic reduction—and, for that, medicine plays an important role.

If many of the medication options work the same, how do you know which one to choose?

It's often suggested that choosing the right medication among similar ones is like throwing darts at a board. And while it's true that within a given class of medications there is probably no clear "wrong" or "right" suggestions, we like to think that science and clinical experience play critical roles. We look at results from the published literature, previous medication experiences your child may have had, interactions with other medications your child is taking, and other variables, including pharmacokinetics, pharmacogenetics, ability to swallow pills, compliance, and age. We may also explore how effective and well-tolerated medications have been in other members of the immediate family. Finally, we rely heavily on our experience with other patients to inform decision-making. But most importantly, you have to feel confident in your provider's assessment, judgment, and experience because above all else, this is what drives the medication recommendation.

My friend's child takes a specific type of medicine for the same thing and they are happy; can we have that one, please?

It's always interesting to learn from other people's experiences with medicine but every case is truly unique to the individual. Friends' success with particular treatments won't predict your success. One caveat is that sometimes siblings and other first-degree family members respond well to the same treatment based on shared underlying genetics. The same goes for side effects—just because a friend or even sibling had a negative reaction to a particular medicine does not mean your child will.

If genetics are so important, why don't you just use those genetic tests?

While genetic testing to determine a particular response to a medication (i.e., pharmacogenetics) offers much promise, the translation into clinical practice has been slow and not yet as widely useful as we would have hoped. In the current state, pharmacogenetic testing may help predict tolerability in a small subset of patients who have variations in their liver enzyme genes that are responsible for metabolizing medications. These genetic variants may lead an individual to be a slow or ultra-rapid metabolizer of certain medications and this could justify using very low doses (for slow metabolizers) or high doses (for ultra-rapid metabolizers). But the reality in working with children is that we should always *Start Low and Go Slow* until we see benefits based on the clinical presentation. Doses can be increased based on the need for benefits or decreased based on the presence of side effects. While reports from pharmacogenetic testing companies may make claims that certain genetic profiles (i.e., gene variants) may predict response to certain medicines, the evidence for this remains very limited at present. With more genetic testing and results from more studies, however, these claims may eventually materialize.

So genetic testing is good for nothing?

Not nothing, but we do not recommend them from the outset. They can be helpful in predicting tolerability to medicine and may explain why your child needs very low or high doses. So sometimes they can be useful if finding the right medicine is especially challenging.

I'm pretty convinced the medications are safe, but how effective are they?

The answer will be different for each medication (and for every child), and we will include discussions of effectiveness in all the following subsections.

All right, we picked one, now how do I talk to my kid about this?

The answer to this question depends in large part on the age of the child and where they are in their development. Most children and adolescents can identify issues that they acknowledge are challenging for them—anger, sadness, anxiety, impulsivity, getting frustrated easily, difficulty focusing, restlessness, etc. It can be helpful to link the use of medicine to improving symptoms the child themself identifies. This conversation should be direct and specific. It is important for the child to understand that these are just symptoms and do not define them or imply they are not worthy, competent, or valued in general. Remind them that people take medicine for all kinds of reasons—asthma, diabetes, allergies—and medications for emotional health are no different from medications for physical health. We generally think it's important for the provider to first introduce this discussion so they are the ones "giving" the medicine, not the caregiver. Setting up this dynamic can be helpful for various reasons, including opening up a line of communication directly between your child and the provider. Also, just in case your child may be likely to refuse to take the medicine, being thoughtful about this dynamic from the outset can sometimes avoid power struggles—yes, we're familiar with the rare possibility that you and your child may engage in power struggles on occasion . . .

Why are my child and their older sibling on the same dose if they are so much smaller?

Children exhibit differences in the pharmacokinetic properties of medications; understanding this is fundamental to prescribing. Pharmacokinetic properties include the absorption, distribution, metabolism, and elimination of a medication, and each of these elements is impacted by age. Oral *absorption* of a medication in children may be affected by gastrointestinal maturation and the prevailing microbiome. Body composition of water and fat also varies with age leading to differences in how medication gets *distributed*. In addition, compared to adults, children have a greater liver-to-body-weight ratio and differences in the levels of liver enzymes, which affect medication *metabolism*. Finally, children have higher filtration rates through the kidneys, leading to faster *elimination* of certain medications.

But that is not true for all medications, right? Because I hear from their pediatrician that many medications are dosed by weight.

It is true that some medications have guidelines for prescribing that are based on weight, especially in pediatric populations (e.g., antibiotics, growth hormone). And while the doses in FDA registration trials in child psychiatry are in part selected based on weight, fixed dose ranges are generally used when medications become commercially available. Regardless, child psychiatrists should always *Start Low and Go Slow* according to clinical symptoms and side effects. With a few exceptions, we rarely use weight-based dosing paradigms.

Can we cut the pills if we need to in order to give the right dose?

Always check with your provider or the pharmacist before you cut pills. As a general rule, cutting "long-acting" or "extended-release" formulations of medications should be avoided because it disrupts how the medicine is delivered and acts on the body. "Immediate-release" forms of medicine, on the other hand, may come in tablet forms that are "scored" for easy splitting. The "score" is the indented line that runs across the surface of some tablets that make them easy to split in half.

How long after starting medication will we see improvement?

The answer to this important question depends heavily on the medication and the individual and their sensitivities. Because we *Start Low and Go Slow*, we generally prefer to ensure safety first, even if it takes longer to see benefits. With some medications, benefits can be immediate (i.e., day 1), and with others, it can take weeks to even months. We will provide more specific answers to this question in the following chapters.

If my child is struggling with more than one condition, how should we approach this?

We hear you—kids are very complicated and often going through lots of developmental changes all at once. Unfortunately, co-occurring conditions are all too common—we call this "comorbidity." In these cases, we find it most helpful to prioritize symptoms and try to approach one at a time. Sometimes many different symptoms, even across conditions, can improve with one medication. At other times, two different medications may eventually be needed, but it's safest to start one at a time or else it can be challenging to figure out which is helping or causing side effects.

Our provider said our child might need more than one medicine; is this common?

Co-occurring conditions, or comorbidity, is indeed common and often requires more than one medication. Under these circumstances, your provider should be able to explain how the medications act differently on the body (i.e., pharmacodynamics) and why more than one is needed to address the various symptoms. A common concern raised by caregivers is when providers use a second medicine to treat the side effects of the first medication. We definitely get how this causes a philosophical twitch and can lead to questioning the whole endeavor of medicating your child. Generally this approach can be avoided by reducing or changing the medicine that causes the side effects. However, sometimes it takes several medication trials to find the right medicine, or combination of medicines, and upsetting this gentle balance can lead to a recurrence of symptoms. For example, if you finally found a medicine to treat your child's rip-roaring case of ADHD and they are doing well in school after years of struggling, you may be willing to use a second medicine to address the subsequent sleep problems likely caused by the ADHD medicine before risking a recurrence of symptoms by making broader changes.

What about therapy instead of medicine— isn't this a safer approach?

Therapy can be extremely helpful, depending on the child and the condition, and most psychiatric disorders in children and adolescents are best treated with a combined approach. Empowering a child to understand the nature and extent of their symptoms and to adopt techniques to improve coping is extremely helpful, especially in the long term. In some conditions, awareness and implementation of effective strategies can even replace the need for medicine over time. However, in conditions like ADHD, bipolar disorder, and psychotic illness, medication is necessary and considered the first-line of treatment. In others, like depression and OCD, their use is typically reserved for moderate to severe cases. As providers, we have a toolbox of interventions and will discuss all of them with you. For children, we often want to apply every tool we know is safe and effective to ensure the child stays on, or returns to, a healthy developmental trajectory. The long-term consequences of not doing everything possible may be profound, and like you, we all want what's best for our kids.

How about exercise, diet, and a good sleep schedule?

As with all behavioral health conditions, proper sleep, hygiene, healthy diet, and, ideally, exercise are a pre-requisite for well-being but do not replace the need for appropriate treatment with medicine and therapy.

Where can I find out more about medications?

Not Wikipedia or Dr. Google please. We strongly advise developing a relationship with a knowledgeable provider whom you trust and who can communicate effectively and clearly. This person will be responsible for prescribing medicine to your child and needs to be able to make you and your child feel confident in their abilities. The internet is filled with conflicting advice and misinformation, and it is very difficult for parents to discern reliable resources. As such, we advise that the first and primary resource should be your provider; ask them for additional materials so you can also do research on your own. The American Academy of Child and Adolescent Psychiatry also offers some excellent online resources for parents and caregivers to learn more about psychiatric medications (www.aacap.org).

My insurance never wants to pay for the brand name medicine—is generic fine?

Generic medications are required by law to have the same active ingredients as the original brand form. However, they may not necessarily be as potent, and some generic versions can be as much as 10 percent less potent than the brand equivalent. This difference may result in a given dose feeling less effective, and therefore sometimes (but rarely) dose adjustments are required when switching between brand and generic versions, or even between different generic versions of medications. In addition, some of the inactive ingredients (i.e., excipients) may be different between brand and generic versions and this could lead to new side effects in a minority of people who are very sensitive to generally benign substances that are used to promote stability, absorption, or solubility of medications. Finally, generic versions may look and taste different from brand versions and, while this does not affect its benefit, it's important to be aware of it.

My provider is an expert but has been involved in many clinical trials sponsored by drug companies; do they have a conflict of interest?

This is always an important question to ask your provider to assess potential conflicts of interest. There is also a national database where this information is publicly available according to the Sunshine Act (https://openpaymentsdata.cms.gov). A full list of our disclosures appears in the appendix.

Chapter 4

Attention-Deficit/Hyperactivity Disorder (ADHD) Medications

What is ADHD really and doesn't everyone have it?

ADHD is one of the most common psychiatric conditions in pediatric populations, with an estimated frequency of 6 percent worldwide. ADHD is characterized by symptoms of inattention and/or distractibility or hyperactivity and impulsivity. Obviously these symptoms affect all children and adolescents (and adults too), but we don't consider them to meet criteria for ADHD unless they are especially severe (typically more severe than 90 percent of the population), occur across at least two settings (e.g., home and school), and create significant impairment in daily functioning. Fortunately, the safety and benefit of medications as a first-line treatment for ADHD is strongly supported in the literature based on decades of research.

What are the main medications used to treat ADHD and how do they work?

There are two main classes of medications used in the treatment of ADHD: (1) stimulants and (2) non-stimulants, including (2a) norepinephrine reuptake inhibitors and (2b) alpha-2 receptor agonists. ADHD symptoms are generally thought to arise from dysregulation of dopamine and norepinephrine chemical systems that operate across brain networks, including in the front part of the brain called the prefrontal cortex. The prefrontal cortex is responsible for executive

Nerve Cell
Figure 2

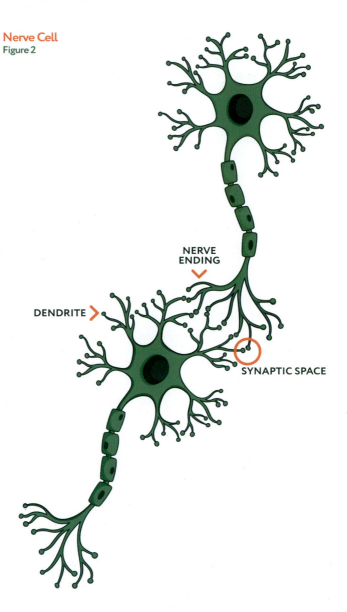

NERVE
ENDING

DENDRITE

SYNAPTIC SPACE

functioning, like attention, organizing, sequencing, and planning. Brain imaging studies have shown differences in the structure and function of the brain across regions responsible for attention, emotion regulation, and motor activity in people with ADHD as compared to people without ADHD. These symptoms are caused by complex changes in the regulation of several chemical systems and nerve cell networks spread across multiple brain regions. Medications are meant to improve regulation of the chemical systems and refine communication between nerve cells (figure 2). While there is interplay between many different chemical systems in the brain, the medications we use to treat symptoms of ADHD mainly target dopamine and norepinephrine.

The following section will review how the different medications used to treat symptoms of ADHD are thought to work. This is generally called the *mechanism of action*.

SECTION 4A

Mechanism of Action of ADHD Medications

STIMULANTS

There are two groups of stimulant medications, those derived from amphetamines (e.g., Adderall) and those derived from methylphenidate (e.g., Ritalin). Stimulants increase dopamine and norepinephrine activity through multiple mechanisms. Both groups of medications block the dopamine transporter, which serves to regulate how much dopamine is taken up back into the cells. When the dopamine transporter is blocked, it effectively increases the amount of dopamine available to be released between nerve cells (figure 3). So yes, blocking the dopamine transporter essentially increases levels of dopamine available to pass between nerve cells. Stimulants also work very quickly. In fact, the first day your child is on an effective dose, they will experience benefits. Unfortunately, stimulants do not reach a steady state, so their effect wanes by the end of the day, and "every day is a new day" as we say. This also means that in the morning before the medicine takes effect and at the end of the day after the effect is gone, your child may experience

Stimulants
Figure 3

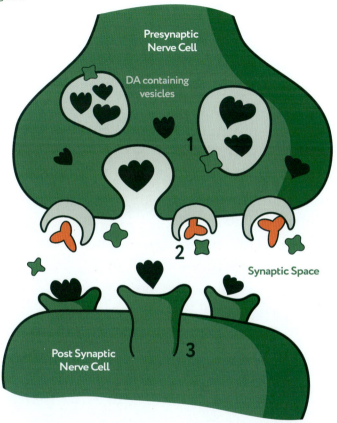

1 AMP increases release of DA from presynaptic vesicles.

2 AMP and MPH block DA reuptake transporters and increase release of DA into the synapse.

3 Increased nerve cell transmission of DA.

 Dopamine (DA)

DA transporters

 DA receptors

Amphetamine (AMP)

Methylphenidate (MPH)

Norepinephrine Reuptake Inhibitors
Figure 4

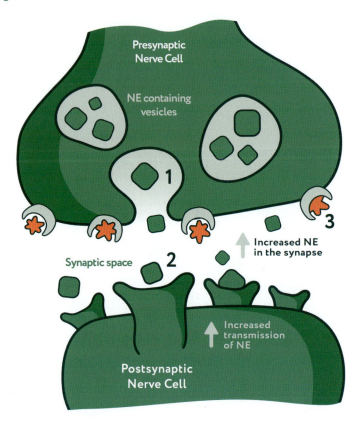

Presynaptic Nerve Cell

NE containing vesicles

Synaptic space

Increased NE in the synapse

Increased transmission of NE

Postsynaptic Nerve Cell

- Norepinephrine (NE)
- NE transporters
- NE receptors
- Strattera

1 NE is released into the synapse.

2 NE attaches to receptors.

3 Strattera blocks reuptake of NE from the synaptic space.

difficulties. This is during times when they still may need the benefit of the medicine (getting ready for school in the morning and doing homework in the evening), but there are strategies to avoid these ups and downs, which we'll review in more detail later in this chapter.

NOREPINEPHRINE REUPTAKE INHIBITORS

Norepinephrine reuptake inhibitors (e.g., Strattera and Qelbree) are *non-stimulants* that block the reuptake of norepinephrine transporters and are relatively selective for the transporters in the prefrontal cortex. Norepinephrine reuptake receptors in the prefrontal cortex are also sensitive to dopamine. So, the net effect of this class of medication is to increase levels of norepinephrine, as well as dopamine, mainly in the prefrontal cortex (figure 4). Recall that the prefrontal cortex is like a command center of the brain responsible for critical things like attention and impulse control; norepinephrine and dopamine drive communication between nerve cells in the prefrontal cortex that serve these functions. Norepinephrine reuptake inhibitors can take weeks to fully work. While there is a subset of kids who respond to very low doses, medicines like Strattera and Qelbree require patience as the concentration accumulates over time. Repeated doses, given either once or twice a day, allow the medicine to reach a steady state and eventually produce the downstream changes in regulation of norepinephrine and dopamine that is associated with the benefit. The advantage of the non-stimulants is that because they reach a steady state, they are always providing benefit and there should not be the "on/off" effect that is seen with stimulants.

ALPHA-2 AGONISTS

Alpha-2 agonists (e.g., Intuniv and Kapvay) are also *non-stimulants* that have a complicated mechanism of action but—to put it in overly simplified terms—they act on different alpha-2 receptor subtypes to also regulate levels of norepinephrine and dopamine (figure 5). These receptors are present in the prefrontal cortex, among other brain regions, so we imagine you're starting to see the theme here. Like norepinephrine reuptake inhibitors, alpha-2 agonists require repeated dosing over weeks to achieve the desired effect.

Alpha-2 Agonists
Figure 5

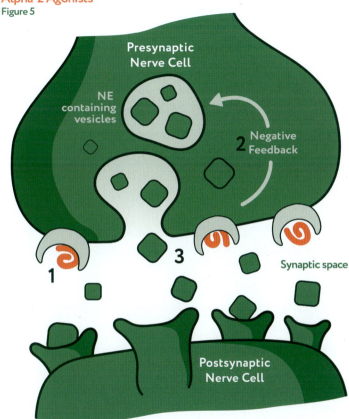

Presynaptic Nerve Cell

NE containing vesicles

2 Negative Feedback

3

Synaptic space

1

Postsynaptic Nerve Cell

- Norepinephrine (NE)
- Alpha 1 receptor
- Alpha 2 receptor
- Intuniv

1 Alpha-2 Agonists activate presynaptic alpha-2 receptors.

2 Alpha-2 receptors are inhibitory and their activation stimulates negative feedback.

3 The net effect is to reduce the release of NE.

SECTION 4B

Evidence for the Use of ADHD Medications

Stimulants have strong evidence to support their use in the management of ADHD, with similar efficacy and tolerability across amphetamine and methylphenidate compounds and all are FDA-approved across a wide range of ages. Adderall, for example, is an amphetamine approved in children down to three years old. Ritalin is a methylphenidate compound approved in children from the age of six, but approval parameters do not mean there isn't significant evidence of safety in younger children. While some providers may be reluctant to use medicine to treat younger children with ADHD, depending on the individual circumstances and severity of symptoms, it may be important to at least carefully consider it. Adverse consequences on self-esteem and feeling a lack of self-competence and self-control can already start to take hold in very young children; intervening early can have enormous social, emotional, and academic benefits. Indeed, the Preschool ADHD Treatment Study (PATS) examined the effect of Ritalin in 303 preschoolers, aged three to five-and-a-half years (Greenhill et al., 2006) and found significant improvement as compared to the placebo.

TABLE 2. AMPHETAMINE-BASED STIMULANT MEDICATIONS FOR ADHD

MEDICATION (GENERIC NAME)	FORMULATION	AGE
Adderall (amphetamine/ dextroamphetamine)	Tablet	≥3
Adderall XR (amphetamine/ dextroamphetamine)	Extended-release capsule	≥5
Adzenys XR (amphetamine)	Extended-release, orally disintegrating tablet	≥6
Dexedrine (dextroamphetamine)	Extended-release capsule	≥6
Dynavel XR (amphetamine)	Extended-release tablet	≥6
Evekeo (amphetamine)	Tablet	≥4
ProCentra (dextroamphetamine)	Liquid	≥3

MEDICATION (GENERIC NAME)	FORMULATION	AGE
Vyvanse (lisdexamfetamine)	Extended-release capsule	≥6
Zenzedi (dextroamphetamine)	Tablet	≥3

TABLE 2A. METHYLPHENIDATE-BASED STIMULANT MEDICATIONS FOR ADHD

MEDICATION (GENERIC NAME)	FORMULATION	AGE
Aptensio XR (methylphenidate)	Extended-release capsule	≥6
Contempla XR (methylphenidate)	Extended-release, orally disintegrating tablet	≥6
Daytrana (methylphenidate)	Transdermal (on skin) patch	≥6
Jornay PM (methylphenidate)	Extended-release capsule	≥6

MEDICATION (GENERIC NAME)	FORMULATION	AGE
Focalin (dexmethylphenidate)	Tablet	≥6
Focalin XR (dexmethylphenidate)	Extended-release capsule	≥6
Methylin (methylphenidate)	Liquid	≥6
Quillichew ER (methylphenidate)	Extended-release, chewable tablet	≥6
Quillivant XR (methylphenidate)	Extended-release liquid	≥6
Ritalin (methylphenidate)	Tablet	≥6
Ritalin LA (methylphenidate)	Extended-release capsule	≥6

Norepinephrine reuptake inhibitors also have multiple studies to support their use to treat symptoms of ADHD. Both Strattera and Qelbree are approved in children as young as six years old. While effective and well tolerated overall, the percentage of people who respond to norepinephrine reuptake inhibitors and the magnitude of the response is likely lower than with stimulants. This compromise may be worth it, however, when you consider the benefit of a medicine that reaches a steady state and provides benefit consistently throughout the day.

Alpha-2 agonists are also approved for the treatment of ADHD, including as adjunctive therapy, meaning in combination with stimulants. Both Intuniv and Kapvay are approved in children from six years old and have evidence from rigorous studies demonstrating their benefit. The consensus among providers, however, is that alpha-2 agonists are more effective in treating hyperactivity and impulsivity than inattention. In addition, alpha-2 agonists are commonly and effectively used to treat tic disorders and Tourette's disorder, which can co-occur with ADHD.

TABLE 3. NON-STIMULANT MEDICATIONS FOR ADHD

MEDICATION (GENERIC NAME)	FORMULATION	MECHANISM	AGE
Strattera (atomoxetine)	**Extended-release capsule**	**Norepinephrine reuptake inhibitor**	$\geqslant 6$
Qelbree (viloxazine)	**Extended-release capsule**	**Norepinephrine reuptake inhibitor**	$\geqslant 6$
Catapres✥ (clonidine)	**Tablet**	**Alpha-2 agonist**	$\geqslant 6$

MEDICATION (GENERIC NAME)	FORMULATION	MECHANISM	AGE
Kapvay (clonidine)	Extended-release tablet	Alpha-2 agonist	⩾6
Tenex* (guanfacine)	Tablet	Alpha-2 agonist	⩾6
Intuniv (guanfacine)	Extended-release tablet	Alpha-2 agonist	⩾6

*off-label use only

Knowing the mechanism and all the research is great, but will the medication work in my child?

Stimulants are among the most-effective medications we have in child psychiatry. About 70 percent of kids will respond and show improvement in symptoms of inattention, hyperactivity, and impulsivity. Response rates to non-stimulants are lower, but they are still effective and come with advantages over stimulants in terms of more sustained benefit throughout the day and potentially fewer side effects, which could include appetite suppression and sleep disturbance.

SECTION 4C

Contemplating Using ADHD Medications

Aren't there, like, a million different kinds of stimulants?

Yes and no. All the stimulants are either amphetamine- or methylphenidate-based. In other words, all are basically forms of either Adderall or Ritalin.

What are the main differences between stimulants?

The differences mainly revolve around how stimulants are packaged into capsules or tablets and the way they are delivered over the course of the day, which determines duration of the effect. For example, Concerta is a long-acting form of methylphenidate that uses an osmotic pump embedded within the capsule to release methylphenidate slowly and usually lasts about ten to twelve hours. Adderall XR (extended-release), on the other hand, packages amphetamine as little beads into a capsule. As the capsule absorbs water in the gut, about half of the beads burst, releasing amphetamine. The other half of the beads are timed to release later because they have a thicker coating and require more water to be absorbed before bursting. Adderall XR is essentially a double-pulse mechanism that is ideally meant to last up to twelve hours, but often lasts closer to eight hours. Vyvanse has an especially interesting delivery mechanism; an amino acid called lysine is attached to the amphetamine molecule and only after the lysine gets cleaved using proteins in the gut does the active form of the amphetamine get released. These lysine components are cleaved as the drug travels though the gastrointestinal system, slowly releasing amphetamine throughout the day, ultimately lasting ten to fourteen hours. Other forms of amphetamines (e.g., Evekeo) and methylphenidates (e.g., Ritalin) are considered "immediate-release," where the medicine is packaged into a simple tablet that gets absorbed through the gut quickly and lasts about four to six hours.

As you can predict, sometimes using immediate-release forms of stimulants are helpful for the evening in order to complete homework after the extended-release stimulants wear off. The challenge, of course, is to time the dosage in a way that helps maximally but doesn't disrupt dinner or sleep.

Matters are further complicated by the fact that every chemical molecule has left and right sides of their structure that are mirror images of each other. Called enantiomers, they are usually labeled simply as "left" or "right" or some fancy medical term in Latin indicating the same (e.g., dextrorotatory and levorotatory). Sometimes only one side of the molecule is mainly the active one and sometimes both sides are necessary to produce the therapeutic effect. Ritalin, for example, consists of both the right and left side of the methylphenidate molecule, whereas Focalin is only the right side. Similarly, Adderall consists of both sides of the amphetamine molecule, whereas Dexedrine is only the right side.

The differences between stimulants are really complicated; how do you choose?

Hopefully you don't choose and your provider does. Just in close collaboration with you. This gets back to the importance of doing a thorough assessment to understand your child's individual needs. The timing of the greatest challenges throughout the day, baseline issues around appetite and sleep, ability to swallow pills, and many other factors go into deciding which stimulant is right to start with your child. Choosing the right formulation requires deep knowledge of the mechanisms and extensive experience, but in most cases, it is possible to find a safe and effective dose.

Would you ever just start with a non-stimulant?

There are significant advantages of non-stimulants over stimulants. While stimulants work relatively quickly and the magnitude of the effect is often bigger, non-stimulants reach steady-state levels in the system and are therefore always helping your child throughout the day. You avoid the "on/off" phenomena that you see with stimulants and can minimize the notorious challenges in early mornings and evenings when stimulants are typically not working. It is also common to prescribe both stimulants and non-stimulants together for this reason. During the day, when your child needs the benefit the most, the combination provides the most robust effect. In the evening and morning, they may do well enough with just the effect of the non-stimulant. It is also commonly the case that non-stimulants are better tolerated, especially for kids with underlying anxiety. There are fewer risks on the heart, less appetite suppression, and less sleep disturbance than often seen with stimulants.

What are the alternatives?

There are always alternatives to medicine. In treating ADHD symptoms, it is critical to organize the academic and home environments in ways that help compensate for the deficits. Clear expectations, simple directions, structured environments, and frequent breaks are just some examples of techniques that can help kids (and adults) meet their full potential. Many excellent books have been dedicated to outlining behavioral and academic strategies for children with ADHD. However, with ADHD, it is clear that optimal outcomes are achieved with the combination of medication and behavioral interventions. ADHD is biologically based and needs a treatment that addresses the underlying biology.

However, medications also do not replace the need for academic support, healthy diet, or exercise, for example. Digital therapeutic devices have also gained increased attention; in 2020, the FDA approved the first game-based digital therapeutic to improve attention in children with ADHD, called EndeavorRx. In general, choosing treatment is always about weighing risks and benefits, and while the risks of various alternative treatments are likely low, if not zero, the benefits are not nearly as robust as with traditional medications.

Can't diet and exercise do the same thing as stimulants?

Diet and exercise are critical for mental and physical well-being. Healthy food choices and physical activity can certainly improve symptoms of inattention and hyperactivity, but diet and exercise alone will not be adequate to treat ADHD and should not replace the need for medicine.

Why does it slow down my child if it is a stimulant?

The idea behind stimulants and why they work with hyperactivity is confusing and somewhat counterintuitive. One predominating theory is that kids with ADHD actually have lower levels of dopamine at baseline and generally tend to have a sluggish cognitive tempo. This underactivity contributes to their constant need for movement and stimulation. It also accounts for why only highly rewarding activities like sports or video games sustain their attention. Stimulants work by increasing levels of dopamine, thereby helping kids stay focused, even on more mundane tasks. They get bored less easily and have a reduced need for movement and activity. The medications may also engage the "brakes" of the brain in the prefrontal cortex, slowing down movements and improving impulse control.

Aren't you giving medications to treat an external problem?

ADHD symptoms are considered biologically based and occur as a result of changes in chemical regulation in the brain. While external factors can clearly exacerbate symptoms, they are not considered to be the "cause" of ADHD in any given case. That said, environmental changes, such as educational accommodations (e.g., sitting in the front of class, extra time on tests, or taking exams in settings free from distraction), can improve symptoms of ADHD.

Does my child really need this?

ADHD is associated with a multitude of adverse developmental outcomes. If left untreated, ADHD can increase the risk for academic challenges and possibly school failure, substance abuse, interpersonal conflict, and even motor vehicle accidents, among other problems. The mainstay of treatment for ADHD includes stimulants and non-stimulants, and if effectively treated, these risks are reduced.

Would you put your kid on it?

Yeah, we would. Experts in the symptoms and treatment of ADHD should be familiar with the decades of rigorous research clearly demonstrating the efficacy of stimulants, the mitigation of risks such as school failure and substance abuse, and the improved long-term functional outcomes. As such, we would put our children on stimulants or non-stimulants to treat ADHD if indicated.

Are they on it for life?

Assuming the benefits outweigh the risks, most kids elect to continue treatment for as long as they are in an academic setting. However, with natural brain development over time, symptoms often improve, even if they don't entirely remit, and the need for medicine may become less critical as they age. More often than not, the child will be the one to decide whether or not they want or need the benefit of medicine, and hopefully this is a collaborative discussion that occurs between them and their provider. Ideally, the decision to stop or reassess the need for medicine is made with close consideration of the risks of not treating ADHD. It is well-established that ADHD is associated with increased risks, including on relationships and work performance, which proper treatment mitigates. At the same time, many people with ADHD learn what the best life circumstances are, professionally and personally, to help them overcome their symptoms that make medicine less critical.

Do people "outgrow" ADHD?

ADHD is now known to be a lifelong illness for most people. Although symptoms of hyperactivity and impulsivity can improve significantly over time, inattentive symptoms typically persist. While it is true that many adults learn how to compensate for the challenges they face as a result of having ADHD, the need for medicine depends on the severity of symptoms, the extent of work and interpersonal impairment, and often the type of job they have. Many adults learn to develop appropriate support in the workplace or choose work that is highly structured. For example, people with ADHD often are highly creative and have the "big ideas," but they are challenged when it comes to paying attention to the details and executing the ideas. As such, putting support teams in place can compensate and obviate or reduce the need for medicine. Others prefer to take it on an "as needed" basis in high-pressure situations or if deadlines are looming. Others still prefer to take it daily because ADHD also affects day-to-day functioning and relationships.

Is it addictive or habit forming?

There are several components of "addiction" and only some are relevant to treatment with stimulants. While the body does not become physiologically "dependent" on stimulants, most experience a recurrence of ADHD symptoms when they are discontinued. And if treatment has occurred over a prolonged period, stopping abruptly can be associated with "withdrawal" or feelings of lethargy in some cases as the body adjusts. This type of lethargy can persist for a day or two but should not occur for longer than a week. In addition, over time, the body may adjust to a given dose of stimulant in a phenomenon known as "tolerance"; it is often the case that doses need to be increased to continue to achieve the same effect over time.

While withdrawal and tolerance may be characteristics of addiction, stimulants are not typically considered addictive. People with ADHD do not generally "crave" stimulants or abuse them when prescribed appropriately. They rarely engage in risky behavior to obtain stimulants or have any difficulty stopping use should they so desire.

Will it change their brain?

Medications are intended to alter the regulation of brain chemistry, so in a literal sense, yes, they will change how the brain functions. In particular, medication can increase dopamine delivery to critical parts of the brain that regulate attention. As a result, brain activation patterns change during cognitive tasks as suggested by increased oxygen levels in specific regions of the brain responsible for executive functioning (e.g., attention, planning, sequencing, memory).

SECTION 4D

Side Effects of ADHD Medications

What are the most common side effects?

As a group, stimulant medications have similar adverse effect profiles. Common side effects include appetite suppression, headaches, nausea, anxiety, irritability, and insomnia. Some people also find it "dulls" them and makes them quieter or more withdrawn. In some cases, it causes increased heart rate and blood pressure, which need to be monitored as you increase the dose.

The side effects from non-stimulants can vary dramatically, depending on the medicine. In general, they may be better tolerated than stimulants. With Strattera, for example, the main risks are nausea, headaches, sedation, and constipation as the individual is getting adjusted. Elevated heart rate and blood pressure can also occur rarely and require monitoring. According to the FDA, there is a risk of suicidal thinking with Strattera and Qelbree, but—while important to take very seriously—it is quite rare. See the section on SSRIs for more details on the risk for suicidal thinking and behavior.

The side effects of the alpha-2 agonists mainly relate to risks of *decreased* heart rate and blood pressure that requires monitoring. Sedation is possible also, as are headaches. And if one stops alpha-2 agonists abruptly, there is a risk of rebound hypertension.

Will it stunt their growth?

Stimulants certainly suppress appetite and it's important to monitor height and weight routinely. While historically there was some concern about growth suppression, today it appears pretty clear that if there is any loss to height, it is no more than about one-half inch. Skipping doses on weekends, holidays, and during summer breaks is often a good way to maintain body weight and support healthy growth patterns. We recommend taking the medicine during or after breakfast before the appetite suppressing effects take hold. Some decrease in appetite during the day when the medicine is working fully is probably inevitable. And then, as the medicine wears off toward the end of the day, appetite is restored—sometimes with a vengeance!

Non-stimulants are not associated with any significant growth suppression.

Will it affect puberty?

Stimulants or non-stimulants do not delay or promote pubertal onset.

Will it affect their heart?

Cardiovascular effects include a small increase in heart rate and blood pressure, which requires monitoring. Stimulants like amphetamines and methylphenidate have historically been thought to increase the risk of heart problems, including sudden cardiac death. However, a definitive study published in 2011 in the *New England Journal of Medicine* concluded that there was "no evidence of increased risk of serious cardiovascular effects among children and young people who use ADHD medications." Notably, this study was conducted in more than 1.2 million children over more than 2.5 million person-years of follow-up and found only seven serious cardiovascular events that occurred, a rate no greater than the general population risk. Nevertheless, if there is a family history of someone having a heart attack at a young age or any known heart problems in your child, we recommend getting an electrocardiogram (EKG) and echocardiogram before starting stimulants.

Will it change their personality?

Some people complain that stimulants can make them feel "quieter" or "withdrawn" or can subdue some of the "silly" aspects of their personality. These effects can contribute to a sense of "dulling" their personality. Other people are at risk of feeling more anxious or irritable. While these are considered significant side effects, they occur in a minority of people. And for many, these side effects diminish as people get accustomed to the medicine over time. In those for whom these unpleasant side effects persist, however, the effects are entirely reversible and don't continue after the medicine is stopped. Generally speaking, personality changes are an indication to consider changing medicine. Not all stimulants affect people in the same way, so changing the type of stimulant (e.g., from a methylphenidate to an amphetamine-based compound) or the delivery mechanism (e.g., from a capsule to a skin patch) can make a big difference in tolerability.

The experience of taking non-stimulants is often subtler and associated with fewer side effects of feeling "withdrawn" or "quieter," especially after people get adjusted. People who take non-stimulants do not usually complain about feeling as though their personality is changed.

Will it make them a zombie?

Stimulants are rarely associated with sedation, and it's typically sedation or lethargy that can appear "zombie-like." Non-stimulants can cause some initial sedation that can be minimized if the provider makes sure to *Start Low and Go Slow*. If sedation occurs, it should not last more than a week or two and should wane slowly as your child adjusts to the medicine. If your child seems overly sedated, it's definitely an indication to decrease the dose or switch medicine.

Will they lose creativity?

Some people with ADHD are highly creative and the experience of having ADHD can lead to a flooding of ideas with limited ability to filter out the "noise" and enhance the "signal." As a result, effectively treating these symptoms should improve focus, enhance attention to detail, and facilitate successful completion of tasks. At the same time, however, this experience of "flooding" may diminish and feel like a loss of creativity. As always, the risks must be balanced by the benefits. In some cases, people elect to retain their experience of having lots of ideas, perhaps at the same time, even if it means having difficulty executing any of them.

What do you do if there are side effects?

Many side effects of stimulants improve as people get adjusted. For those side effects that don't improve, careful consideration of risks weighed against benefits must be given. Some risks are clear "deal-breakers" and warrant immediate discontinuation. For example, extreme irritability or anxiety, horrible headaches, and total insomnia need not be tolerated for any period of time. There are so many different ways to formulate and deliver stimulants that it is often the case that switching the type of stimulant or delivery mechanism can reduce side effects while retaining benefits.

SECTION 4E

Logistics of Using ADHD Medications

How long will it take to work?

With stimulants, effects can occur within forty-five minutes to an hour after receiving the appropriate dose. Doses are partly weight-based, but once the correct dose is achieved, the benefit is virtually immediate. Side effects are also likely to occur immediately. However, while benefits are typically sustained with continued use, many side effects diminish within one to two weeks.

With non-stimulants, full effects can take weeks, even months, depending on how quickly you can reach a therapeutic dose.

How will we know if it's working?

The effect of stimulants can be pretty dramatic, and often teachers and parents will describe improved focus, longer duration of focus, and decreased hyperactivity and impulsivity almost immediately. With non-stimulants, effects can be more gradual and subtle and take longer to manifest. Some children can clearly describe the benefits, but other children may be unaware or unable to describe the changes they feel. Often the same parent- and teacher-rating scales done during the initial assessment are used to monitor improvement, and you can see numerical changes in scores, improved school performance, and possibly even better handwriting as evidence that the medicine is working.

Can they skip weekends?

Maybe! For some, symptoms are manageable outside of the academic environment and taking breaks on weekends, holidays, or over the summer is perfectly reasonable. Taking brief breaks from stimulants can also prevent tolerance from developing and serve to sustain benefits at a given dose and keep doses at the lowest possible level. Non-stimulants, on the other hand, need to be taken consistently. In fact, stopping abruptly can be associated with discomfort. With alpha-2 agonists specifically, stopping abruptly can cause rebound hypertension and should be avoided.

How do you know what dose to give?

Doses are based first on tolerability, then on effect. Our practice is typically to *Start Low and Go Slow*, increasing doses as tolerated, until the desired effect is achieved. Dosing is also guided in part by weight, where doses of stimulants can be as high as one to two mg/kg/day depending on the stimulant and individual tolerability. The maximum dose of Strattera is approximately 1.4 mg/kg/day according to the FDA label, but there are safety data at higher doses (up to 1.6 mg/kg/day up to a maximum of 100mg/day). Dosing is also determined by past clinical trials in patients and toxicology studies in animals. The FDA reviews all these studies and provides dosing guidelines that are published on the label.

How long will the medicine stay in their system?

The length of time a given medicine will stay in the body is determined by a variety of factors, the most important of which is its half-life. The half-life is defined as the amount of time required for most people to clear half of the medication from their system (Table 1). Liver and kidney function, urine acid balance, and the amount of fat tissue a person has all contribute to the elimination rate of medication. For amphetamines, the half-life is around ten hours, while for methylphenidate, the half-life is much shorter, around three-and-a-half hours. It is important to understand that with stimulants, the duration of the medicine's effect on the body (pharmacodynamics) is dissociated from the time it takes to clear the medicine out of the system (pharmacokinetics). For non-stimulants like Strattera, the half-life is typically about five hours, but once daily dosing still results in sustained effects. Guanfacine is an alpha-2 agonist that has a much longer half-life of around seventeen hours and is typically given once daily (extended-release formulation—Intuniv) to twice daily (immediate-release formulation—Tenex). Clonidine has a half-life as short as five hours and should be given twice daily (extended-release formulation—Kapvay) or three times a day (immediate-release formulation—Catapres) for optimal effects.

What happens if my child drinks alcohol or smokes when they're taking medicine?

For adolescents and young adults, drinking alcohol, smoking (nicotine or marijuana), and vaping are common and important issues to consider. While we generally caution against alcohol- and drug-use, it is important to be realistic about relatively typical teenage activities. While there are clear risks of substance use, particularly for people with ADHD and other psychiatric problems, it is not medically dangerous when stimulants and non-stimulants are used in prescribed doses with moderate amounts of alcohol, nicotine, or marijuana. That said, it is likely that kids will be more vulnerable to the effects of drugs and alcohol while taking stimulants, may feel the effects of drugs or alcohol more quickly, or may experience the effects as more unpleasant. As such, even greater caution is necessary in counseling about the risks of drugs and alcohol while taking psychiatric medications in general.

SECTION 4F

Monitoring ADHD Medications

How often will we need to come in?

The frequency of appointments depends on a variety of factors, the most important of which is how well your child is doing. Different providers have different practice styles, and many prefer to see patients weekly, or at least monthly, until symptoms have improved significantly and the medicine dose is stable. Because stimulants are considered "controlled" substances according to the Drug Enforcement Agency, refills are prohibited. As a result, many providers feel most comfortable seeing patients monthly when each renewal must be prescribed. Nonstimulants, however, can be prescribed with refills. Common practice would dictate that patients are seen at least every three months when stable.

Do they need to see the cardiologist?

Stimulants and atomoxetine can increase heart rate and blood pressure and both need to be monitored routinely. For people with a family history of heart problems at young ages (e.g., heart attacks in people under sixty), it is necessary to get an EKG and possibly an echocardiogram to make sure there is no underlying heart problem before starting stimulants. Stimulants can increase the risk of heart problems in people who have underlying structural defects (e.g., "holes" in the heart) or arrhythmias (electrical conduction or heart rhythm problems). EKGs and echocardiograms are both benign and non-invasive procedures and, while it is not specifically recommended, there is little risk in being cautious and doing the exams either before or early on in treatment with stimulants. Ongoing monitoring should be performed by your psychiatric provider unless the cardiologist indicates otherwise.

Can we stop it abruptly?

There is no need to slowly decrease stimulants before stopping. While a slow taper may reduce the risk of withdrawal lethargy, it is not dangerous to stop abruptly. With the norepinephrine reuptake inhibitors, withdrawal symptoms like anxiety are rare, but it may be safest to taper slowly out of an abundance of caution. As noted, the alpha-2 agonists should be decreased slowly to avoid rebound hypertension.

Do we need to get blood work done to monitor these medications?

Routine annual monitoring during regular check-ups with your child's pediatrician is adequate unless there are specific concerns. Generally this should include an assessment of kidney and liver function and will be sufficient.

Chapter 5

Antidepressant and Antianxiety Medications

What are the main medications used to treat depression and anxiety and how do they work?

Antidepressants and antianxiety medications generally act by regulating three different neurochemical systems critical for mood and anxiety states: serotonin, norepinephrine, and dopamine. Their effect is to block the reuptake of these chemicals back into cells, causing an initial net increase and eventually adjusting the sensitivity of the relevant chemical receptors and triggering the release of various growth factors. These growth factors are thought to promote new nerve cell growth. There are many different classes of antidepressants and dozens of individual agents. By convention, antidepressants are grouped by their main mechanism of action.

SECTION 5A

Mechanism of Action of Antidepressant and Antianxiety Medications

Tricyclic antidepressants (TCAs) were the first class to be introduced and generally target all three main chemical systems: serotonin, norepinephrine, and dopamine. The mechanism of action of TCAs is multifaceted but all block serotonin and norepinephrine reuptake transporters. However, TCAs have an affinity for multiple other chemical systems in the brain leading to many "off-target" effects and are associated with side effects like dry mouth, blurred vision, dizziness, sedation, urinary retention, constipation, and weight gain. Tricyclic antidepressants are known to be highly effective, but because of their side-effect profile, they are rarely studied or used in children and adolescents. One notable exception is Anafranil, which is FDA-approved to treat OCD in children down to ten years old. Despite TCAs' effectiveness in treating depression and anxiety disorders, they have been largely replaced by newer and better-tolerated medications, such as selective serotonin reuptake inhibitors and serotonin and norepinephrine reuptake inhibitors.

Selective serotonin reuptake inhibitors (SSRIs) are the most-commonly prescribed antidepressant and antianxiety medications in children and adolescents. They act by selectively blocking the reuptake of serotonin into cells and cause a net increase in serotonin levels leading to a complicated downstream cascade of cellular events that eventually helps to regulate the brain's serotonin system.

Serotonin and norepinephrine reuptake inhibitors (SNRIs) work similarly to SSRIs and TCAs, but they are selective for both the serotonin and norepinephrine systems. Individual medications in this class have varying degrees of serotonin and norepinephrine activity, which can also be dose-dependent. Importantly, because there are complex interactions between all three chemical systems, SNRIs have been found to also increase dopamine in the prefrontal cortex.

There is another relatively unique antidepressant called Wellbutrin that works by selectively blocking the reuptake of both norepinephrine and dopamine into cells. Wellbutrin is mainly viewed as an antidepressant and, in part because it lacks strong serotonin activity, does not effectively treat anxiety. Regardless, Wellbutrin is rarely used in children and adolescents because there are no FDA approvals for any indication in children and there is a paucity of studies to support its use in pediatric populations.

Antidepressants and Antianxiety Medications
Figure 6

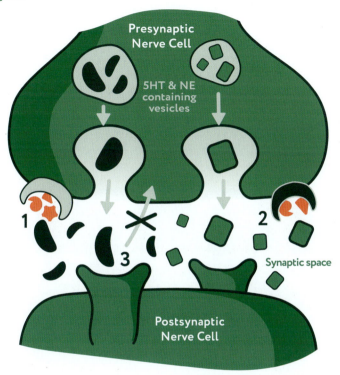

Presynaptic Nerve Cell

5HT & NE containing vesicles

Synaptic space

Postsynaptic Nerve Cell

- Norepinephrine (NE)
- Serotonin (5HT)
- 5HT Transporter
- NE Transporter
- Tricyclic antidepressant (TCA)
- Selective serotonin reuptake inhibitor (SSRI)
- Serotonin and norepinephrine reuptake inhibitor (SNRI)

1 SSRIs selectively block the 5HT transporter to prevent reuptake of 5HT.

2 SNRIs and TCAs block reuptake of both 5HT and NE.

3 Reuptake blockade increases the concentration of 5HT and NE in the synaptic space and enhances nerve cell transmission.

Evidence for the Use of Antidepressant and Antianxiety Medications

Antidepressants have documented efficacy in the treatment of childhood depression, anxiety disorders, and OCD. We will focus on antidepressant medications with indications in pediatric populations, which include SSRIs and SNRIs. In addition, we will briefly review TCAs, which can be useful in the treatment of anxiety disorders and OCD.

It is very important to emphasize that, as a general rule, antidepressants and antianxiety medications are used in conjunction with therapy. Clinical trials also generally demonstrate that the combination of medicine *and* therapy is superior to either alone to treat depression and anxiety.

How effective are the medications?

There is robust and conclusive evidence that medicines like SSRIs are effective at treating depression and anxiety in children and adolescents. Numerous studies provide support for their use across a range of conditions, including major depressive disorder, generalized anxiety disorder, and OCD. Response rates may vary dramatically depending on the individual, but there are many options among the antidepressant and antianxiety medications that, in all likelihood, your provider can find a medicine that helps significantly.

Anxiety disorders often co-occur with each other and have similar symptoms across diagnostic categories. They also often respond to the same medication in a given individual. Examples of anxiety disorders include generalized anxiety disorder, social anxiety disorder, selective mutism, panic disorder, separation anxiety disorder, and phobias. However, it should never be the case that two medications in the same class are used together to treat different anxiety disorders in the same person. It would not be appropriate, for example, to use one SSRI to treat generalized anxiety and a second SSRI to treat social anxiety. Because of the commonalities across anxiety disorders and the high degree of response to similar medications, they will be collectively referred to here as anxiety disorders.

Many studies have demonstrated the efficacy of SSRIs for the treatment of anxiety disorders, including Zoloft, Prozac, Luvox, Celexa, Lexapro, and Paxil. At least two SNRIs—Effexor and Cymbalta—also have evidence to support their use in treating children and adolescents. Results from trials with TCAs for anxiety disorders in children and adolescents are mixed; given their side-effect profiles, TCAs are usually reserved for treatment-resistant cases and need to be used cautiously.

The most severe form of anxiety is probably OCD, which luckily responds well to antianxiety medication, and several

SSRIs (Prozac, Zoloft, Luvox) have FDA approvals to treat OCD in children. However, in cases where SSRIs or SNRIs are not adequately effective, at least one TCA—Anafranil—can be highly effective. In fact, Anafranil was the first FDA-approved medication for the treatment of OCD in children (1998).

Two SSRIs—Prozac and Lexapro—have FDA approvals to treat depression (i.e., major depressive disorder) in children and adolescents. Prozac is approved in children as young as eight years old and Lexapro is approved in children from twelve years old. In addition, virtually all of the SSRIs and SNRIs, as well as some TCAs, have been studied in children with depression, but results overall are mixed.

TABLE 4. COMMON ANTIDEPRESSANT AND ANTIANXIETY MEDICATIONS

MEDICATION (GENERIC NAME)	FDA INDICATION	MECHANISM	AGE
Anafranil (clomipramine)	Obsessive-compulsive disorder	TCA	⩾10
Celexa (citalopram)	n/a[a]	SSRI	n/a
Cymbalta (duloxetine)	Generalized anxiety disorder	SNRI	⩾7

MEDICATION (GENERIC NAME)	FDA INDICATION	MECHANISM	AGE
Lexapro (escitalopram)	Major depressive disorder	SSRI	≥12
	Generalized anxiety disorder		≥7
Luvox (fluvoxamine)	Obsessive-compulsive disorder	SSRI	≥8
Paxil (paroxetine)	n/a	SSRI	n/a
Norpramin (desipramine)	Major depressive disorder	TCA	≥13
Prozac (fluoxetine)	Major depressive disorder	SSRI	>8
	Obsessive-compulsive disorder		>7
Wellbutrin (buproprion)	n/a	NDRI[b]	n/a
Zoloft (sertraline)	Obsessive-compulsive disorder	SSRI	≥6

[a]n/a = not applicable (i.e., not FDA approved in children)

[b]NDRI = norepinephrine and dopamine reuptake inhibitor

SECTION 5C

Contemplating Using Antidepressant and Antianxiety Medications

So we know antidepressant and antianxiety medicines work, but are they safe?

The medicines used for anxiety and depression have been used for decades; the first medicine—Prozac—was approved for the treatment of depression in adults in 1987 and in kids in 2003. SSRIs and SNRIs are generally well tolerated. Common side effects include nausea and headaches. For some people, SSRIs and SNRIs can make them feel drowsy, while others can feel more alert or "activated" and have difficulty sleeping. Antidepressants can also cause restlessness, mood fluctuations, and even increased anxiety early in treatment. As mentioned already, TCAs can have a range of additional side effects, including dry mouth, blurred vision, dizziness, and urinary retention; they are typically avoided (except for treating OCD) in children and adolescents for this reason.

The vast majority of side effects with antidepressant and antianxiety medications can be managed symptomatically, like taking a Tylenol to avoid headaches or taking the medicine with food to avoid nausea. If it makes your child drowsy, they can take it at night. And if it makes them alert and causes sleep disturbance, they can take it in the morning. Most side effects should go away as your child adjusts over the first few weeks of treatment. If side effects don't get better, or at least become manageable, this likely indicates the need to adjust the dose or change medicine.

Can antidepressant and antianxiety medications make my child worse?

For all antidepressants, there is a small risk of developing symptoms that are essentially on the opposite extreme of depression, called "mania" or "hypomania." This is a risk for a small subset of vulnerable people, including those with a family history of bipolar disorder. For this reason, the initial assessment should include a thorough family history. Antidepressant use always necessitates close monitoring of mood, energy, and sleep, among other side effects.

What's the story with antidepressants causing people to commit suicide?

Since 2004, all antidepressants have an FDA-issued black box warning indicating increased risk of "suicidal thinking and behavior" in people under twenty-five years old. This warning was issued on the basis of a large study that combined data from twenty-four studies (called a meta-analysis) with antidepressants across 4400 participants. Results suggested that among participants who received active treatment with an antidepressant in these studies, the risk of suicidal thinking was 4 percent. Among participants who received a placebo, on the other hand, the risk was 2 percent. While not clinically meaningful (the difference between 2 and 4 percent), it was statistically significant. It should also be noted that none of the participants in the trials completed suicide. Nevertheless, these results led directly to a warning for all the antidepressants in people under twenty-five years old. Unfortunately, this warning also led to a reduction in prescription rates, by as much as 50 percent according to some studies, and there was a subsequent increase in suicide rates. Even more unfortunate is that today, suicide is the second-leading cause of death among teenagers.

What are the alternatives? Can't diet and exercise do the same thing? What about CBD?

There are always alternatives, including no treatment at all. Short of a judge mandating treatment, taking medications is always voluntary. For depression and anxiety disorders, SSRIs are unequivocally the first-line treatment. This is because they are generally effective and well tolerated. Diet and exercise are also crucial, of course. For some, regular exercise can minimize or potentially even replace the need for medications. Homeopathic remedies and nutraceuticals (sometimes called alternative or complementary medicine) can have a role as well. The challenge with these medications (yes, they're medications too) relate to the industry's regulation. Whereas conventional medications like SSRIs must first prove they are safe and effective before becoming commercially available, herbal supplements are assumed to be safe. They get stocked on the shelves of pharmacies and health food stores and are only removed if shown to be unsafe, often after millions of people have already consumed them. There is also the possibility that the supplement may not actually be what you think it is. For example, a tablet you think consists of one milligram of melatonin may actually be fifteen milligrams of Chinese sawdust. And not the good kind.

CBD and its various forms may hold promise, but more studies are needed, especially in children, before we would feel comfortable making assessments of its effectiveness and safety.

Does my child really *need* medicine to treat their depression and/or anxiety?

It's important to understand that medicine for depression and anxiety is not curative, but it does reduce symptoms effectively and safely. Your child doesn't have to take Motrin for a headache, but if they do, they will probably feel better. They may not *need* Prozac for depression or anxiety, but if their symptoms are causing significant distress and impairing their ability to socialize or get to school, we think it's important to provide all of the tools we know can help. In some cases of severe distress, there is even suicidal thinking, and medicine may play an important role in reducing the risk of suicide.

Aren't you giving medications to treat an external problem?

We think of depression and anxiety as occurring because of a complex interplay between biology (e.g., genes) *and* the environment (figure 7). In other words, you could expose ten kids to the same environmental stressor and only those who are biologically vulnerable will experience depression or anxiety. And while environmental stressors can exacerbate symptoms, for many kids, depression and anxiety often feel like they occur for no particular reason and seem to come "out of the blue." Changing the environment is certainly a key to helping symptoms. Supportive school environments and parent training are undoubtedly helpful. Like psychotherapy, the environment can also fundamentally alter brain function and should be addressed as part of treatment. However, sometimes medicine is also warranted to address the underlying biological vulnerability, especially if symptoms are so severe or functioning is so impaired that your child can't meaningfully engage in therapy.

Biopsychosocial Model of Depression and Anxiety
Figure 7

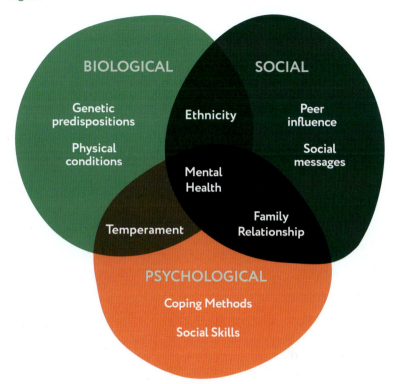

Is medicine just a band-aid that masks the underlying problem?

Sometimes medicines are certainly viewed this way; in our view, this is in part because of ongoing stigma about mental illness. We see medications as an important tool that provides significant symptomatic relief, which in turn can allow therapy to help. Medicine helps facilitate behavioral changes where insight and effective coping strategies can really take hold.

Do you always recommend medications?

Giving your child medication for depression or anxiety is always a very challenging decision to make. Sometimes parents feel as though they have somehow failed if their child needs medicine. Sometimes there is grief associated with the "loss" of a healthy child and taking medicine highlights the extent to which the child is suffering. There are typically three categories into which this discussion with your provider falls. One, the advice is that medicine is not necessary so either the symptoms should be monitored before intervening or the child should start with some form of psychotherapy. Two, the recommendation is made strongly to start medicine because the child is suffering immensely and, in combination with therapy, we want to apply every tool possible to address their distress. Ongoing depression and anxiety can be quite debilitating and associated with major problems in school, at home, and socially. Depression is also associated with increased risk of suicide, a devastating and tragic outcome. The third category in this discussion is likely the most common and one where you may or may not decide to start medicine and you collaborate with your provider to carefully discuss all risks and benefits and consider the timing of starting medicine, if at all. The circumstances surrounding the symptoms are critical here, as are the extent, severity, and duration of symptoms. It is important to note that

FOR ANXIETY AND DEPRESSION

individual attitudes play an important role; some families have very positive, even life-changing, experiences with loved ones taking medicine, whereas others want to avoid using medicine to the extent possible.

Would you put your child on it?

Based on our decades of experience, we have had the opportunity to see remarkable and life-altering effects with antidepressant and antianxiety medications. From our perspective, the vast majority of children benefit from these medicines and few have unpleasant side effects. Sometimes the first medicine tried isn't effective or well tolerated, but there are many, many options, so it is very likely that with patience and time, your provider will find a medicine that significantly helps your child. While concerns about risks and skepticism about benefits may be warranted, these medicines are globally safe and effective. Any concerns are mainly theoretical unless and until the medicine is tried. After a trial, you will be in a better position to fully judge the risks and benefits. Because side effects of antidepressants and antianxiety medicines are mainly unpleasant but not dangerous, and because none of the side effects last long after you stop, we encourage a trial if you're contemplating. Only then will you fully appreciate the effects, good and not so good. In short, if one of our children was suffering from debilitating depression or anxiety, we would not hesitate to use medicine.

How long will they be on it for?

This is a great question and one with no specific or consistent answer. The general consensus is to wait about six to twelve months after symptoms resolve before slowly stopping medicine. The caveat is timing. If the one-year mark falls just before the SATs, that is probably not an ideal time to come off a medication. We typically wait until a low-key time, such as summer break. Even then, if your child will be away from home over the summer, this may not be ideal. You can see how this gets complicated in the lives of busy kids. We promise the intent is not to keep your child on medicine forever and this is not a conspiracy by pharmaceutical companies to boost profits. With discussion, you and your child's provider will be able to find an appropriate window of time to stop medicine slowly with minimal risks.

Is it true there is "withdrawal" and it's really hard to stop the medicine?

Some people indeed experience side effects coming off antidepressant and antianxiety medications. This is sometimes referred to as "withdrawal" or a "discontinuation syndrome" and is usually avoided by decreasing the medicine slowly. These side effects can include flu-like symptoms, insomnia, nausea, dizziness, sensory disturbances (e.g., "tingling" or "electric shock-like" sensations), and increased anxiety or irritability. Yes, we know that sounds terrible, and while it can be, it occurs in a minority of people and is not medically dangerous. Some of the medicines are worse offenders than others in this regard and this variability depends, in part, on the elimination rate. In the same way that we *Start Low and Go Slow* when we begin treatment, we also stop medicine slowly. How slowly depends on the individual and the medicine (i.e., pharmacokinetics), but a general rule is to reduce the dose by about 25 percent per week. This tends to minimize any unpleasant withdrawal effects in the vast majority of people. In those for whom withdrawal persists, we'll say again that, while uncomfortable and unfortunate, it is short-lived and *not* medically dangerous.

Is the medicine addictive?

There are always fears that kids will become "dependent" on medicine or that they will never be able to stop because their body will continue to need it. Or even worse, the fear that symptoms will be even worse after attempting to stop because somehow brain chemistry has been permanently altered. Typical antidepressants or antianxiety medicines can only be considered "addictive" in the sense that in some cases doses need to be increased over time to sustain effects (i.e., tolerance develops), and that if stopped abruptly, withdrawal symptoms like worsening anxiety can occur briefly. For this reason, it can feel unpleasant to have to rely on taking medicine every day and fear-provoking to forget medicine while away for the weekend or on vacation. However, antidepressants and antianxiety medicines are not addictive in that people don't abuse or misuse them and stopping (slowly) is always possible. Sometimes symptoms return upon stopping, but these are underlying symptoms re-emerging as the effects of the medicine wanes, not a sign of being "addicted."

There is a class of antianxiety medicines called benzodiazepines (e.g., Ativan, Klonopin, Xanax, Valium) that are more addictive in the traditional sense of the term. Higher doses are gradually needed to achieve the same effects and dependence develops relatively quickly (within weeks), so if stopped abruptly, it can cause very uncomfortable anxiety and even seizures in some cases after long-term use at relatively high doses. Benzodiazepines are very effective for short-term use or intermittent use on an as-needed basis only. They are sometimes prescribed to kids for extreme anxiety or sleep disturbance in the context of a death in the family, divorce, or major life transitions. Children with anxiety disorders can also briefly use benzodiazepines while they wait for the benefit of more traditional SSRIs to take effect, which is often a matter of several weeks or even longer. We also use benzodiazepines for kids with neurodevelopmental disorders, like autism spectrum disorder, to treat severe aggression or self-injury.

Will it change their brain?

As discussed, antidepressants and antianxiety medicines work by blocking the reuptake of chemicals—serotonin, norepinephrine, and dopamine—in brain cells. These chemicals play critical roles in regulating mood and anxiety states. The medicines essentially make more of these chemicals available to the brain and thereby change brain chemistry and brain function. Brain structure is not otherwise affected and, after your child stops medicine, the chemistry reverts back to its baseline state. However, the way our brain functions also depends on how we perceive and process information, so positive changes that occur under the influence of medicine and therapy can sustain themselves beyond the treatment period.

SECTION 5D

Side Effects of Antidepressant and Antianxiety Medications

What are the side effects and how will I know if my child is having them?

Usually if you have to be looking hard for them, they're not there. We feel comfortable prescribing these medications because they tend to have few side effects. The most common side effects are probably on the gastrointestinal system because antidepressant and antianxiety medicines mostly affect serotonin, and serotonin receptors are even more abundant in the gut than in the brain. These side effects can include stomachaches, nausea, rarely vomiting, and diarrhea or constipation. Yup, why the same medicine can cause constipation and diarrhea is confusing, and we don't have a good explanation except to say that it's usually one or the other in a given person, not both. Ditto for sleep-related side effects. Some people feel drowsy and others have trouble sleeping. Vivid dreams can also happen, as can excessive sweating, especially at night. Another relatively common side effect is headaches, and some people complain about dry mouth.

Do these medications cause sexual side effects?

Annoyingly, some people can have sexual side effects. This may be decreased sex drive (libido), erectile difficulties, or delays in the time it takes to orgasm. These side effects are much more common in adults than teenagers, but it's still very important to discuss. In our view, problematic sexual side effects can be a reason to stop or switch medicine, and sometimes reducing the dose can also help.

What about weight gain?

Weight can either go up, down, or stay the same, depending on the person. Excessive weight gain is rare, but people who gain weight while on the medicine may have more difficulty losing weight while continuing the medicine. Weight and appetite should be monitored, and if unwanted weight gain occurs and it is hard to lose, this may also be a reason to stop, change, or reduce the medicine.

Can we talk about the black box warning again?

When the SSRIs hit the market in the late 1980s and early '90s, there was excitement because they were very helpful and well tolerated. Finally, there were medicines to help kids with depression and anxiety! Unfortunately, kids with depression are at increased risk for suicidal thinking and suicide in general, and soon after these medicines started being widely prescribed, anecdotal reports and small case studies of increased suicidal thinking after starting antidepressants began to emerge. While two events that occur together does not mean that one *caused* the other, these reports were important to take seriously and led to very large studies to evaluate the risk. We also know that kids with depression are already more likely to have suicidal thoughts, and kids with depression and suicidal thinking are more likely to require antidepressants, so we needed to be certain that antidepressants were not causing harm. Despite the fact that completed suicides did not appear to increase, results from the FDA analyses were concerning enough to lead the agency to issue a black box warning that all antidepressants, when used by people under twenty-five years old, may cause an increased risk of "suicidal thinking and behavior." Since this time (2004), it's become clear that there were several flaws in the analytic methods, and the FDA warning may have actually caused harm because providers stopped writing prescriptions for antidepressants to kids who needed them. It may not be a coincidence that while mortality rates for teens have steadily decreased since then, suicide rates have increased and, by 2014, suicide replaced homicide as the second-most common cause of death among teens.

Nonetheless, your provider should regularly be asking your child about suicidal thoughts. Current guidelines for initiating antidepressants in children suggest monitoring weekly for the first month, biweekly for the next month, and then monthly. This risk is one of the major reasons we *Start Low and Go Slow*, but we feel strongly that the benefits of antidepressant and antianxiety medications generally outweigh the risks.

Will it change their personality or make them a zombie?

Medicine should not change your child's personality, and if there are signs of dulling or decreased "spark" or feeling less talkative or creative, the medicine should be adjusted or changed altogether. Some people report feeling emotions less intensely while on the medicine and this may actually be perceived as a benefit. For some, however, it feels unsettling, so a risk/benefit analysis is appropriate to decide whether to continue, change, or stop altogether. While the benefit of reduced panic or crying episodes may be robust, for example, the risk of feeling emotionally "dulled" may not feel worth it. Again, it is important to understand that these side effects do not occur in most people, and when they do occur, they are typically short-lived (one to two weeks) or addressed through subtle manipulations of the dose or timing of the medicine.

Will it stunt their growth or affect puberty?

Antidepressants and antianxiety medicines do not affect growth or puberty. In some cases, children may have increases or decreases in appetite, which may warrant weight monitoring. These effects are not common, however, and tend to be insignificant and easily managed.

SECTION 5E

Logistics of Using Antidepressant and Antianxiety Medications

How long until we see symptoms improve?

The answer varies a lot and depends on the person and the individual circumstances. Some people say they start feeling better almost immediately. For most, it's between two and six weeks. Some really don't see benefits until twelve weeks on the medication, so it usually makes sense to stick with it—assuming any side effects are tolerable. Even worse for those of us who love instant gratification, recent studies have shown maximum benefit may not even occur until twenty-four weeks.

How will we know if it's working?

There should be both subtle and obvious signs the medicine is working to reduce your child's distress and improve their functioning. It is very important to establish clear, measurable, and realistic target symptoms you are looking to see improve

KOLEVZON, JAFFE, AND TRELLES

by using medicine. Whether panic, crying, school refusal, or irritability, there should be symptom reductions that are evident to you (as a caregiver), other relatives, and even teachers. Your child may be able to also describe the benefit, depending on their age and emotional maturity. If improvement is not clear, it may be worth slowly stopping to reassess and re-evaluate the effectiveness.

What if my child misses a dose?

Missing one or maybe two doses, depending on the antidepressant, is probably fine. Missing doses should not affect mood, but it may affect anxiety because of the risk of withdrawal symptoms. Antidepressant and antianxiety medications vary in how long they stay in your system, so ones that have longer half-lives and slower elimination times (e.g., Prozac) are much less prone to problems if you skip doses compared to others (e.g., Luvox). If you end up missing doses for more than a few days, speak with your provider because they may decide to restart at a lower dose.

If we miss one dose, should we take two the next day?

No, please don't.

What if it's already the afternoon and we forgot the morning medicine?

No biggie. You can always check with your provider, but usually it's best to take the medicine and then return to the regular schedule the following day.

Can we skip weekends?

No, antidepressants and antianxiety medicine don't work like stimulants and need to be taken every day to work effectively and avoid withdrawal-related side effects.

How do you know what the right dose is?

Unfortunately, we don't. We have a general sense of the minimal effective dose and the maximum dose based on the published research and information provided by the manufacturer, but every child is very different. Generally, we balance wanting to find the lowest possible dose that works and wanting your child to feel better as quickly as possible. At the same time, we often say that if your child is taking medicine, they should be taking a dose that truly helps them. We also know that side effects are sometimes related to how high the dose is and how quickly we increase the medicine. Finally, often times the benefit of a given dose reaches a plateau or underlying symptoms recur and dose increases are required. These factors make prescribing something of an art, in addition to a science.

Are higher doses more effective?

The right dose can vary dramatically between people and across medicines. With the same exact medicine, one person may respond robustly to half the dose of another person. And while some medicines are prescribed using weight-based guidelines, this is not the case for antidepressants and antianxiety medicines. Especially when looking at different medicines, the idea of "high" and "low" dose cannot be compared. Some antidepressants and antianxiety medicines are more potent and therefore five, ten, or fifteen milligrams can be very effective, whereas others are less potent, so doses of one hundred, two hundred, or even three hundred milligrams are needed. The dose does not generally correspond to how "sick" the child is, but instead reflects individual metabolic factors, genetics, and the specific medicine. As a reference, Tylenol is usually taken at 325 milligrams or 500 milligrams, which may sound "high," but this illustrates how comparing doses between different medicines is like comparing apples to oranges. To use a related analogy and reinforce the idea of focusing on the benefit and not the dose: if you had a headache, you wouldn't take half a tab of Tylenol—you'd likely take two.

How long will the medicine stay in their system?

The half-life of antidepressants and antianxiety medicines is highly variable, ranging from about ten hours to up to three days. In most cases, the half-life is long enough that the medicines can be taken once daily and still reach a steady state in the blood.

Can they drink and/or smoke while taking antidepressant and antianxiety medications?

Alcohol and drugs can have serious effects on mood and anxiety states. Alcohol is generally considered a "depressant" and should be avoided in kids prone to depression. Marijuana is commonly used among teens; for those vulnerable to anxiety, marijuana can make it worse, even leading to panic attacks. Some people believe marijuana calms their anxiety, but they may find themselves in a negative cycle of using drugs to self-medicate. The effects of medicines may be counteracted by using drugs and alcohol for the reasons described. Further, side effects from medicines may be exacerbated by drugs and alcohol or you may experience the effects of drugs and alcohol more intensely and more easily when taking antidepressants or antianxiety medicines. The effects of drugs or alcohol may also be different and more unpleasant while taking antidepressants and antianxiety medicines. Finally, benzodiazepines and a rarely prescribed type of antidepressant called MAO inhibitors are quite dangerous to take with drugs or alcohol and should be strictly avoided.

SECTION 5F

Monitoring Antidepressant and Antianxiety Medications

How often will they need to come in?

At first as we *Start Low and go Slow*, your child needs to come in more frequently. As noted, guidelines for starting antidepressants in children suggest they are monitored weekly for the first month, biweekly for the next month, and then monthly. This practice varies by provider, but generally kids are seen often until they feel better and safety is confidently established. Once stable, sometimes visit frequency can be decreased, even to every three months. Monitoring of antidepressants and antianxiety medication can also be accomplished, at least in part, using telehealth platforms. While this can reduce burden for your family and be less disruptive for your child's after-school activities, it can certainly be suboptimal for many kids and we do recommend regular *in-person* visits.

Do they need to see the heart doctor or get regular blood work done?

Heart monitoring is not typically necessary with antidepressants or antianxiety medicine. If significant side effects emerge—for example, palpitations and/or excessive sweating—measuring blood pressure and heart rate will be a routine part of the monitoring by your psychiatric provider. If weight gain or weight loss is suspected, your provider should also be monitoring height and weight and possibly metabolic measurements on bloodwork.

Can I stop it abruptly?

Antidepressants and antianxiety medicines should not be stopped abruptly due to the risk of acute withdrawal symptoms known as a "discontinuation syndrome," which is characterized by a wide array of possible symptoms, including flu-like symptoms, insomnia, nausea, dizziness, sensory disturbances (e.g., "tingling" or "electric shock-like" sensations), and increased anxiety or irritability. See the answer to withdrawal symptoms in section 4c.

Chapter 6

Antipsychotic and Mood-Stabilizing Medications

What are the main medications used to treat psychosis and mood cycling and how do they work?

Antipsychotic medications regulate levels of dopamine in the brain and are thought to reduce psychotic symptoms and, to an extent, aggressive behavior and various mood-related symptoms through this mechanism. Antipsychotic medications are divided into two general classes based on their mechanism: (1) "typical" or "first-generation" antipsychotics mainly block dopamine and (2) "atypical" or "second-generation" antipsychotics block both dopamine and serotonin. We will focus on second-generation antipsychotics and briefly describe the differences between older and newer generations.

The first generation of antipsychotics were used in the 1950s (Thorazine) and the second generation began in 1989 with approval for Clozaril. This new generation was described as "atypical" because of the promise of fewer side effects. Although significant side effects persist with both generations of antipsychotics, with a few exceptions, the second-generation options are much more commonly prescribed today, especially for children and adolescents.

Antipsychotic medications have a long history as the first-line treatment for psychotic symptoms and have been approved to treat schizophrenia (Invega, Abilify, Zyprexa, Risperdal), which is the main psychotic disorder in those under eighteen. In recent years, antipsychotics have also received a number of approvals by the FDA for childhood psychiatric disorders other than schizophrenia, including "irritability and aggression" associated with autism spectrum disorder (Risperdal, Abilify), bipolar disorder (Seroquel, Risperdal, Saphris, Abilify, Zyprexa, Latuda), depression in the context of bipolar disorder (Zyprexa), and Tourette's disorder (Abilify). Approved age ranges vary, but Risperdal is indicated for children as young as five years old with irritability or aggression associated with autism spectrum disorder, Abilify is approved for children as young as six years old for children with Tourette's disorder and autism spectrum disorder, and the rest are approved in children as young as ten to thirteen years old, depending on the condition. In addition, antipsychotics are used to treat severe mood dysregulation, chronic tic disorders, agitation, and disruptive behavior that is resistant to treatment in kids with ADHD, autism spectrum disorder, and/or intellectual disability.

TABLE 5. COMMON ANTIPSYCHOTIC MEDICATIONS

MEDICATION (GENERIC NAME)	FDA INDICATION	CLASS	AGE
Abilify (aripiprazole)	Schizophrenia	Second-generation	≥13
	Mania in bipolar disorder		≥10
	Irritability in autism spectrum disorder		≥6
	Tourette's disorder		≥6

MEDICATION (GENERIC NAME)	FDA INDICATION	CLASS	AGE
Haldol (haloperidol)	Schizophrenia	First-generation	⩾3
	Tourette's disorder		⩾3
	Severe behavioral disorders		⩾3
Invega (paliperidone)	Schizophrenia	Second-generation	⩾12
Latuda (lurasidone)	Schizophrenia	Second-generation	⩾13
	Depression in bipolar disorder		⩾10
Orap (pimozide)	Tourette's disorder	First-generation	⩾12
Risperdal (risperidone)	Schizophrenia	Second-generation	⩾13
	Mania in bipolar disorder		⩾10
	Irritability in autism spectrum disorder		⩾5

MEDICATION (GENERIC NAME)	FDA INDICATION	CLASS	AGE
Saphris (asenapine)	Manic or mixed episodes in bipolar disorder	Second-generation	≥10
Seroquel (quetiapine)	Schizophrenia Mania in bipolar disorder	Second-generation	≥13 ≥10
Thorazine (chlorpromazine)	Severe behavioral disorders	First-generation	≥6 months
Zyprexa (olanzapine)	Schizophrenia Manic or mixed episodes in bipolar disorder	Second-generation	≥13 ≥13

Mood stabilizers were traditionally used in psychiatry to treat bipolar disorder, the main mood-cycling disorder characterized by episodes of mania and depression. Lithium was approved for adults with bipolar disorder in 1970 and was the first-line treatment in children for many years, despite not receiving a formal approval by the FDA for children down to seven years old until 2019. Alternatives to lithium are anticonvulsants, which are also known as anti-epileptic drugs because they were initially developed to treat seizures in children and adults with epilepsy.

Anticonvulsants have become the mainstay of treatment of mood dysregulation and bipolar disorder in children and are generally considered safer than lithium. Several anticonvulsants have received FDA approval to treat bipolar disorder in adults (Depakote, Tegretol, Lamictal), but no formal approvals have yet been granted for children. That said, virtually all of the anticonvulsants used in psychiatry have been FDA-approved to treat children with epilepsy, including those we know are effective for adults with bipolar disorder. Aside from lithium, mood stabilizers are prescribed off-label, although there is robust long-term safety data from epilepsy studies.

TABLE 6. COMMON MOOD STABILIZERS

MEDICATION (GENERIC NAME)	FDA INDICATION (OTHER THAN SEIZURES)	CLASS	AGE
Depakote (divalproex sodium)	n/a	Anticonvulsant	n/a
Lamictal (lamotrigine)	n/a	Anticonvulsant	n/a
Lithium/ Lithobid (lithium carbonate)	Bipolar disorder, mania, and maintenance	Mood stabilizer	≥12

MEDICATION (GENERIC NAME)	FDA INDICATION (OTHER THAN SEIZURES)	CLASS	AGE
Tegretol (carbamazepine)	n/a	Anticonvulsant	n/a
Topamax (topiramate)	n/a	Anticonvulsant	n/a
Trileptal (oxcarbazepine)	n/a	Anticonvulsant	n/a

SECTION 6A

Mechanism of Action of Antipsychotic and Mood-Stabilizing Medications

ANTIPSYCHOTICS

All antipsychotics block dopamine receptors, at least partially. This effect regulates dopamine levels and confers their antipsychotic properties. The newer antipsychotics, known as "atypical" or "second-generation," also modulate serotonin receptors, which is thought to confer additional benefits of mood stabilization and reduce the risks associated with dopamine blockade. However, these second-generation antipsychotics come with more metabolic side effects, including weight gain, increased levels of cholesterol and triglycerides, and an elevated risk of diabetes. There is wide variability across the many antipsychotics in terms of which dopamine and serotonin receptors they affect (there are dozens) and the extent to which they bind to them, but the general mechanisms are as described (figure 8).

Antipsychotics
Figure 8

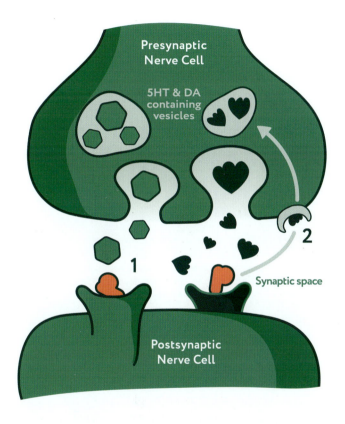

Presynaptic
Nerve Cell

5HT & DA
containing
vesicles

1

2

Synaptic space

Postsynaptic
Nerve Cell

Dopamine (DA)

Serotonin (5HT)

5HT$_{2A}$ Receptor

DA Receptor

Antipsychotics

1 Blockade of DA receptors reduces
DA nerve cell transmission.

2 Second generation antipsychotics
also block 5HT2A receptors to
reduce 5HT nerve cell
transmission.

Mood Stabilizers
Figure 9

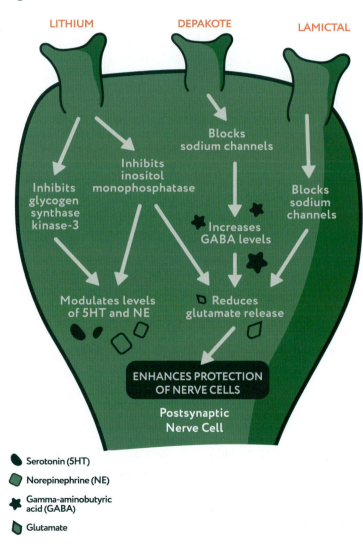

LITHIUM   DEPAKOTE   LAMICTAL

Blocks sodium channels

Inhibits inositol monophosphatase

Inhibits glycogen synthase kinase-3

Blocks sodium channels

Increases GABA levels

Modulates levels of 5HT and NE

Reduces glutamate release

ENHANCES PROTECTION OF NERVE CELLS

Postsynaptic Nerve Cell

Serotonin (5HT)

Norepinephrine (NE)

Gamma-aminobutyric acid (GABA)

Glutamate

LITHIUM

The mechanism of action of lithium is not well-understood, but it likely has effects on several regulatory pathways affecting the communication between nerve cells. In particular, lithium modulates glutamate pathways where glutamate is the primary excitatory chemical in the brain responsible for promoting learning and memory. Too much glutamate, however, can be toxic to nerve cells, so a gentle balance between excitation and inhibition (through another chemical system called GABA) is critical for proper brain functioning. Lithium is also thought to have a protective effect on nerve cells, at least partially, through glutamate-related pathways and stimulating other protective factors, such as brain-derived neurotrophic factor (neurotrophic = nerve growth)(figure 9).

ANTICONVULSANTS

Depakote, Tegretol, and Lamictal are the main anticonvulsant medications with mood-stabilizing properties that we use in child psychiatry. They all work through multiple mechanisms, including regulating excitatory (glutamate) and inhibitory (GABA) activity in the brain by modulating various channels in nerve cell membranes (the layer that separates the interior of the cell from the outside environment), which control communication between cells. Depakote is also thought to have protective effects on the central nervous system by helping promote gene expression and DNA repair, as well as reducing nerve cell death (figure 9).

SECTION 6B

Evidence for the Use of Antipsychotic and Mood-Stabilizing Medications

How effective are the medications?

Next to stimulants, antipsychotics and mood stabilizers are among the most powerful medicines we have in child psychiatry. However, because of their side-effect profile, they should be reserved for serious conditions like psychosis, bipolar disorder, severe OCD, or extreme irritability and aggression. Nearly 70 percent of children with irritability and aggression in the context of autism spectrum disorder respond to antipsychotic medications like Risperdal and Abilify. These same studies also provided evidence for the benefit in treating hyperactivity, motor movements (stereotypies), and repetitive behaviors in autism spectrum disorder. Another common indication for using antipsychotics in children is tics and Tourette's disorder; at least six placebo-controlled studies document their efficacy. Three antipsychotic medications have FDA approval for Tourette's disorder, two first-generation (Haldol, Orap) and one second-generation (Abilify), but several others have been shown to work well depending on the individual (Risperdal, Zyprexa, Seroquel, Geodon). Nevertheless, because of their favorable side-effect profile, the alpha-2 agonists commonly used to treat ADHD are often considered the first-line treatment for tics and Tourette's disorder. Many other antipsychotics have been extensively studied with robust evidence to support their efficacy across a wide range of conditions.

Mood stabilizers like lithium and anticonvulsants are likewise highly effective. Even if mainly prescribed off-label (besides lithium), there are numerous rigorous studies and case reports documenting the efficacy of mood stabilizers to treat bipolar disorder and mood dysregulation in general, disruptive behavior in the context of ADHD and conduct disorder, and aggression. In general, mood stabilizers have fewer side effects than antipsychotics; however, depending on the individual, they may also be less effective. It is not uncommon to take a combined approach in relatively severe cases where a single medication is either inadequately effective or poorly tolerated. Topamax, for example, is an anticonvulsant that is generally well tolerated and has been used effectively to treat bipolar disorder and disruptive behaviors in children. Topamax has a unique side-effect profile that includes appetite suppression, so combining it with an antipsychotic can be a useful strategy to enhance the benefit and reduce the weight gain associated with antipsychotics.

SECTION 6C

Contemplating Using Antipsychotic and Mood-Stabilizing Medications

Do they really need this?

Thinking back to the three categories of discussion (see page 98) about whether to start medicine, if antipsychotics or mood stabilizers are being considered, it is very likely that your child needs to start medicine—perhaps urgently. While the risk profiles of antipsychotics and mood stabilizers can vary and may be significant, the benefit typically outweighs the risk, so the recommendation to start should be taken very seriously.

Would you put your kid on it?

We would reluctantly, and after much careful consideration, allow our children to take antipsychotics or mood stabilizers if warranted, and especially if other more benign options have been tried and failed.

How long will they be on it for?

As with most psychiatric medication trials, it is generally valuable to reassess the need for medicine after your child has been relatively stable for six to twelve months. Psychosis and bipolar disorder are typically considered chronic and lifelong conditions, so it is likely that your child will continue to require medication. However, often dramatic psychiatric symptoms can occur in the context of major life stressors, developmental changes, and trauma, but after effective treatment for a period of time, medicine may no longer be necessary.

Is it addictive or habit forming?

Antipsychotics and mood stabilizers are not considered in any way addictive and not typically abused. Like with most psychiatric medications, however, they can't be stopped abruptly for risk of withdrawal symptoms. Abrupt withdrawal from antipsychotics can lead to an exacerbation of underlying symptoms and a risk of abnormal muscle movements (dyskinesias). Abrupt withdrawal from anticonvulsants can trigger a seizure in children with an underlying vulnerability to seizures.

Will it change their brain?

Antipsychotics block dopamine and serotonin neurotransmission, so yes, they change brain chemistry and function, thereby reducing symptoms. Mood stabilizers have many different mechanisms and exactly how they accomplish their mood-stabilizing effects are not always clearly known. But neither antipsychotics nor mood stabilizers have effects on brain structure, and the effects they do impart are not sustained for the long term once the medicine is cleared from the system.

SECTION 6D

Side Effects of Antipsychotic and Mood-Stabilizing Medications

What are the side effects, and will I know if my child is having them?

Understanding fully the side effects associated with antipsychotics and mood stabilizers and how these risks will be managed and monitored is an absolutely critical in-depth conversation to have with your provider.

The antipsychotic medications work in part by blocking dopamine, which can cause a wide range of associated side effects, including movement problems known as "extrapyramidal symptoms," like muscle rigidity or muscle contractions, restlessness and slow movements, tremors, and irregular, jerky movements (tardive dyskinesia). While tardive dyskinesia is relatively rare in children, it's especially concerning because with long-term antipsychotic use, it can be permanent. Muscle contractions (dystonia) can be severe in rare cases or when doses are too high and providers do not *Start Low and Go Slow*. Dystonia can be painful, and if it occurs in the throat muscles (i.e., laryngeal), it can block the airway and be potentially dangerous. Thankfully, dystonia is easily treated with Benadryl and, even more thankfully, none of us have ever encountered laryngeal dystonia in children in our many decades of collective practice. Blocking dopamine can also cause increases in a hormone called prolactin, which, when elevated, can lead to breast tissue enlargement, breast pain, and even milk discharge. Common and less dangerous side effects from antipsychotics can include things like sedation, increased appetite, weight gain, nausea, drooling, and constipation. Weight gain can be significant, however, and if not carefully monitored, may increase risk for developing diabetes.

In addition, some antipsychotic medications carry cardiovascular risks, which can include EKG changes (prolonged QTc); decreased blood pressure, especially on standing; and increased heart rate (tachycardia). Blood pressure should be monitored at least annually.

If that's not enough to worry about, antipsychotics can also lower seizure threshold, so they need to be used with caution in people who are vulnerable to seizures or taking other medications that also lower seizure threshold. Finally, some antipsychotics have a risk of suppressing the production of white blood cells that fight infection (neutropenia), so monitoring complete blood counts is necessary at least annually. Clozaril, while rarely used in children, is highly effective for people with schizophrenia who have not responded to other antipsychotic medications. However, Clozaril carries an additional risk of severe neutropenia (agranulocytosis), and complete blood counts are monitored weekly for six months when initiating treatment, then biweekly for six months, and then monthly thereafter if stable.

The side effects of mood stabilizers depend on the specific medication. Our answers will focus on those most commonly used in child psychiatry: lithium, Depakote, Tegretol, and Lamictal.

Lithium may be the most challenging to use because it has what is known as a "narrow therapeutic window." This means that the target range in blood levels is small—low blood levels will not help, then there is a small sweet spot, then higher levels can cause significant side effects. The main serious risks of lithium are reducing thyroid function (hypothyroidism) and impairing kidney function. The adverse effects on the kidney relate to a decrease in the kidney's ability to concentrate urine (nephrogenic diabetes insipidus) and can manifest as excessive urination (polyuria) and excessive drinking (polydipsia). Lithium can also cause weight gain, sedation, nausea, headaches, acne, hair loss, and hand tremors. These risks in general can be limited by our *Start Low and Go Slow* mantra and by close monitoring. Lithium is a type of salt, so risks can be minimized by ensuring your child drinks enough fluid and avoids becoming dehydrated.

Depakote can adversely affect liver and pancreatic function, in addition to causing weight gain, sedation, headaches, nausea, tremors, and hair loss. Depakote is also associated with decreased platelets (thrombocytopenia), which can cause problems with blood clotting. In addition, Depakote can elevate levels of ammonia in the blood (hyperammonemia), which can cause toxic levels of ammonia to build up and result in confusion (encephalopathy). However, hyperammonemia is effectively treated with a dietary supplement—carnitine—which helps eliminate excess ammonia from the system. In females, Depakote can cause multiple cysts on the ovaries (polycystic ovarian syndrome).

Tegretol has a similar array of unpleasant side effects that are typically reduced if you *Start Low and Go Slow*. These include drowsiness, dizziness, nausea, vomiting, constipation, blurred vision, tremors, and dry mouth, among other negative effects. While rare, Tegretol is associated with an increased risk of Stevens-Johnson syndrome, which is a rash that affects the skin and mucous membranes. It often starts with flu-like symptoms and then a painful rash can spread and turn into blisters. Stevens-Johnson syndrome is rare and can be avoided by increasing doses slowly. However, it can also be a medical emergency that warrants immediate attention and, in *very* rare cases, can lead to death. Other rare side effects that require monitoring are a type of anemia (aplastic), where the bone marrow doesn't make enough blood cells for the body to function properly, and agranulocytosis, where the body doesn't make enough blood cells to fight infection. Importantly, Tegretol also interacts with many other medications through its effects on liver metabolism proteins, so it's critical to always check with your provider when taking other medications.

Lamictal tends to be very well tolerated, although it's especially critical to *Start Low and Go Slow* in order to avoid the risk of Stevens-Johnson syndrome. In fact, your provider will follow a very specific protocol, slowly increasing Lamictal every two weeks by very small doses to essentially eliminate this risk. As a result, it may take many months before the benefit with Lamictal is clear. Other side effects of Lamictal include dizziness, headaches, insomnia, nausea, vomiting, diarrhea, constipation, and decreased appetite.

Will it change their personality, make them a zombie, or cause them to lose their creativity?

Antipsychotics and mood stabilizers are the kinds of medicines that people complain cause dulling, cognitive slowing, and sedation; hence, they may appear to change personality. These negative effects may be reduced by decreasing the dose. There are also many different types of effective antipsychotics and mood stabilizers and not all cause the same side effects in a given individual. Changing medication type may alleviate some unwanted effects.

Will it stunt their growth or affect puberty?

Antipsychotics and mood stabilizers are not thought to affect height. Some antipsychotics, like Risperdal, have been associated with breast tissue growth due to elevations of a hormone called prolactin. This growth is called gynecomastia and should be monitored with dose reductions or medication changes as needed. Antipsychotics can also affect the metabolism of sugar and fats and cause obesity, particularly around the truncal/waist area.

Some antipsychotics can alter the balance of growth and sex hormones and affect the progression of puberty. Elevated levels of prolactin in females, for example, can cause temporary loss of menstruation until the medicine is adjusted or changed. Lithium can cause impaired thyroid function (hypothyroidism) that either warrants changing medicine or adding thyroid hormone. Chronically low levels of thyroid hormone can delay pubertal onset, among other complications. A rare but serious side effect of Depakote is a condition called polycystic ovarian syndrome in females, which can cause irregular menses, excess male hormones, and ovarian cysts.

SECTION 6E

Logistics of Using Antipsychotic and Mood-Stabilizing Medications

How long until I see something?

Antipsychotics often work quickly, within one to two weeks or sometimes within days, depending on your child and the required dose. Often early experiences of sedation may be calming and contribute to improved sleep and behavior. Responses to lithium and anticonvulsants usually depend on reaching therapeutic blood levels and, depending on the medication, can be increased relatively quickly. The response to Depakote, for example, can also be seen within one to two weeks. Lamictal, on the other hand, requires a very slow titration often over several months to avoid the emergence of a dangerous rash (Stevens-Johnson syndrome).

KOLEVZON, JAFFE, AND TRELLES

How will we know if it's working?

Symptoms treated with antipsychotics and mood stabilizers tend to be relatively obvious, such as irritability, aggression, or mood cycling. As such, improvements should be readily apparent. Accepting that parents are the experts in their children, providers rely heavily on parent reports to gauge improvement. Speaking with teachers directly or arranging calls between the provider and teachers is also highly informative when appropriate. Some providers also use a variety of rating scales filled out by children, parents, and teachers to assess the extent and severity of symptoms during the evaluation that can be repeated after medication is started to measure improvement.

Can they skip weekends?

Antipsychotics and mood stabilizers should be given consistently and not missed for any period of time. When the decision is made to stop, they should be reduced slowly and carefully to avoid the risk of withdrawal.

Can we skip a dose?

Skipping a dose may be uncomfortable and increase anxiety or cause trouble sleeping in some people. Generally, skipping one dose is not dangerous. For people who are vulnerable to seizures, however, skipping a dose of an anticonvulsant type of mood stabilizer (e.g., Depakote, Tegretol, Lamictal) can potentially trigger a seizure and should be avoided.

How do you know what dose to give?

Like with virtually all medicines for emotional and behavioral health, we *Start Low and Go Slow*. Doses are increased based on tolerability and titrated until a significant benefit is achieved. For the antipsychotics, often very low doses can be effective, and risks typically increase as the dose increases. Dose ranges have been established in clinical trials and serve to guide the provider. With risperidone, for example, typical starting doses are around 0.25 milligrams, but the average dose in trials for irritability and aggression in autism spectrum disorder was 1.8 milligrams daily. For many anticonvulsants, dosing is usually guided by blood levels, in addition to clinical benefit, and varies depending on which anticonvulsant is being used. For lithium, dosing is strictly tied to blood levels (0.6 to 1.2 mEq/L) because of the narrow therapeutic window where higher doses can harm the kidneys.

How long will the medicine stay in their system?

Like with all medicines, antipsychotics and mood stabilizers are metabolized and excreted from the system based on elimination rates that vary according to the specific medicine and pharmacokinetic parameters. Once stopped, the benefit diminishes relatively quickly and symptoms may re-emerge. How long it takes for underlying symptoms to recur, if they do at all, is highly variable and relatively unpredictable. However, symptom recurrence depends more on individual differences than on any specific medication's features.

Can they drink alcohol or smoke?

It is not advisable to drink or smoke while taking antipsychotics or mood stabilizers. Generally speaking, alcohol and other drugs will reduce the effectiveness of the medications. Even nicotine, for example, can reduce blood levels of antipsychotics. At the same time, taking psychiatric medications may make people feel the effect of alcohol and other drugs more quickly and in different, perhaps unpleasant ways.

SECTION 6F

Monitoring Antipsychotic and Mood-Stabilizing Medications

How often will we need to come in?

Careful and consistent monitoring is a critical part of taking antipsychotic and mood-stabilizing medications. Depending on the specific medicine, liver, kidney, thyroid, and pancreatic function need to be assessed, in addition to monitoring fat in the blood (cholesterol and triglycerides) and the risk for diabetes (hemoglobin A1c). For these reasons, people who are psychiatrically stable, and for whom medication changes are not active, should be seen at least every three to six months, depending on the individual and the specific medicine. Active symptoms and medication changes warrant more frequent follow-up appointments. Monitoring plans should be clarified at the outset of starting antipsychotics or mood stabilizers to establish expectations and ensure scheduling availability.

Specifically for antipsychotics, the American Diabetes Association and the American Academy of Child and Adolescent

Psychiatry recommend screening at baseline for personal and family history of diabetes and elevated cholesterol and triglycerides (hyperlipidemia), assessment of current weight/body mass index, blood pressure, fasting glucose, and fasting lipid profile. Body mass index should be monitored throughout treatment; fasting glucose and lipid profile, liver function, hemoglobin A1c, and blood pressure should be monitored annually. Elevations in blood levels of prolactin often occur with antipsychotics but are usually not necessary to monitor unless clinical symptoms emerge (e.g., breast tissue growth, pain, or milk discharge).

Do they need to see the heart doctor?

It is not routinely necessary to see a cardiologist before starting antipsychotics or mood stabilizers or to routinely monitor heart function in children without heart disease. However, some medications in these classes, most notably antipsychotics, can increase the risk of changes in the electrical rhythm of the heart (e.g., QT prolongation) and increase the risk of dangerous cardiac rhythm changes (arrhythmias) in people who are vulnerable at baseline. If there are concerns about cardiac risk at the time of the evaluation, your provider may recommend a consultation with a cardiologist or at least to get an EKG before starting antipsychotics or mood stabilizers. In addition, it is important to ensure that a given antipsychotic does not interact with another medication your child is taking (e.g., SSRIs) to increase the risk of cardiac rhythm changes.

Can I stop it abruptly?

As noted earlier, abruptly stopping antipsychotics or anticonvulsants should be avoided because it can lead to an exacerbation of underlying symptoms, risks of abnormal movements in the case of antipsychotics, or seizures in vulnerable children in the case of anticonvulsants.

Chapter 7

Conclusions

Anything we didn't ask that is important for us to know?

Wow, that was a lot. We think most of what you need to know is covered in this guide. But we also know that people tend to walk out of doctors' offices remembering only about 20 percent of what was said to them. So now you know all the questions to ask—write down the answers! Also ask your provider to give you information in writing so you have it as a reference. Bring someone with you to appointments if necessary—they can also take notes, and two sets of ears are better than one. Obviously we can't usually rely on the kids to listen . . . If you start medication, have the provider write down the details of the titration schedule. And don't leave without a follow-up appointment! We all know how challenging it is to coordinate schedules, especially with those irritatingly busy mental health providers.

Any final words of wisdom?

You are on the right path if you found your way to this book. Hopefully it was better than Google. Staying informed and feeling empowered to advocate for your child and even challenge providers is important. If your provider gets defensive or dismissive, find another provider. Trust and communication are the keys to a successful working relationship. And don't be shy about insisting your prescribing provider also speaks with your child's therapist and teachers—this can provide invaluable information you may not fully appreciate until it's done.

Sometimes finding the right medicine for your child can feel like a long journey. And sometimes we find something that works and is well tolerated on the first try. Be patient; like everything else in parenthood, patience is paramount and there are no "quick fixes" (except perhaps with stimulants for ADHD and snacks for after school). Sometimes we see benefits in days to weeks, sometimes benefits require a complex interplay of medicine, therapy, new parenting strategies, educational accommodations, and other environmental adaptations. Sometimes benefits occur and then plateau or even regress. Sometimes each week can have a few good days and a few not-so-good days. The brain and behavior are very complicated—kids' bodies and brains are constantly growing and changing. What might not be the right medicine for your child at eight years old may work beautifully at fifteen after puberty.

Take ownership over your role as the expert on your child. Trust your instincts as the caregiver and relay all your observations to the provider. We rely heavily on parents—as well as the child, therapists, teachers, and our own observations—to make informed treatment decisions. Trust your instincts about whether the provider is a good fit for your child. We have the privilege of working with children into their adolescence and even adulthood, so this can be a long partnership in some cases. Hopefully the relationship with your provider is a meaningful one filled with growth and success. We know for us, it is an honor and privilege to be able to have an impact on your children's lives.

Finally, be gentle on yourselves as caregivers. Raising children is extremely challenging and the idea of using medicine is a lot to handle! Parenting can be an impossible job and most of us are really doing our best, often under *very* difficult circumstances and at great personal costs. We appreciate the courage it takes to ask for help and even consider medication. For all these reasons, this guidebook is dedicated to the caregiver warriors out there who always fight to give their kids everything and anything they need to be successful.

Appendix

Disclosures

Alex has received research support from the following federal, foundation, and commercial sources: National Institute for Neurological Disorders and Stroke; National Institute of Mental Health; National Institute for Child Health and Development; National Institute for Environmental Health Sciences; National Heart, Lung, and Blood Institute; New York Community Trust Jules and Ethel Klein Fund; Beatrice and Samuel A. Seaver Foundation; Klingenstein Third Generation Foundation; Patient-Centered Outcomes Research Institute; ADNP Kids Research Foundation; Simons Foundation; Autism Science Foundation; Autism Speaks; Eisenberg Foundation; Institutes for Translational Sciences at Mount Sinai; AMO Pharma; Hoffmann-LaRoche; Neuren Pharmaceuticals; Seaside Therapeutics; Curemark; Johnson & Johnson; Neuropharm; Bristol-Myers Squibb; and Eli Lilly. Alex has also consulted with or acted as a scientific adviser to the following foundations or commercial entities: Sherkow Center for Autism, Vencerx Therapeutics, BUILD NYC, Klingenstein

Third Generation Foundation, Therapy Lab, Phelan-McDermid Syndrome Foundation–Spain, Ovid Therapeutics, David Lynch Foundation, ADNP Kids Foundation, Ritrova Therapeutics, CureSHANK, Aelis Farma, Enzymotec, Genentech, Supernus Pharmaceuticals, Amo Pharma, Fulcrum Therapeutics, Third Rock Ventures, sema4, 5AM Ventures, Coronis Neurosciences, LabCorp, Takeda, Acadia, Alkermes, Jaguar Therapeutics, GW Pharmaceuticals, Neuren Pharmaceuticals, Clinilabs Drug Development Corporation, Scioto Biosciences, Biogen, and PYC Therapeutics.

Robert has received research support from Teva and Emalex. Pilar has no potential conflicts of interest to disclose.

About Familius

Visit Our Website: www.familius.com

Familius is a global trade publishing company that publishes books and other content to help families be happy. We recognize that every family looks different and passionately believe in helping all families find greater joy, whatever their situation. To that end, we publish beautiful books that help families live our 10 Habits of Happy Family Life: *love together, play together, learn together, work together, talk together, heal together, read together, eat together, give together,* and *laugh together*. Further, Familius does not discriminate on the basis of race, color, religion, gender, age, nationality, disability, caste, or sexual orientation in any of its activities or operations. Founded in 2012, Familius is located in Sanger, California.

Connect

Facebook: www.facebook.com/familiusbooks
Pinterest: www.pinterest.com/familiusbooks
Instagram: @FamiliusBooks
TikTok: @FamiliusBooks

FAMILIUS

The most important work you ever do will be within the walls of your own home.